Human Papillomavirus

Edited by Rajamanickam Rajkumar

Published in London, United Kingdom

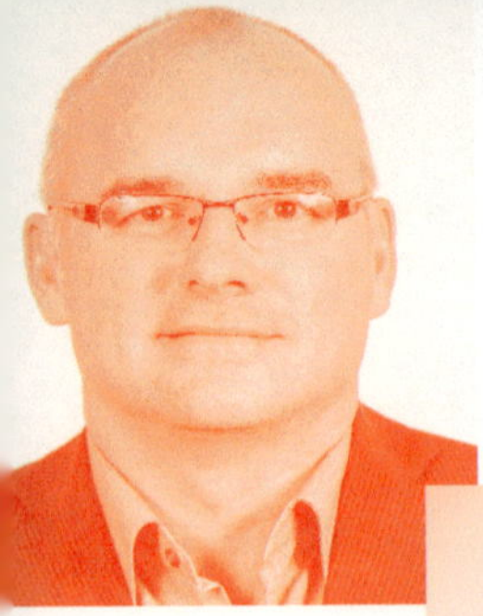
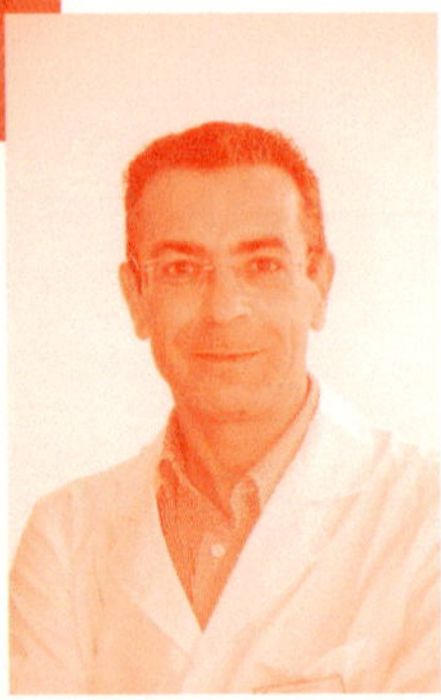
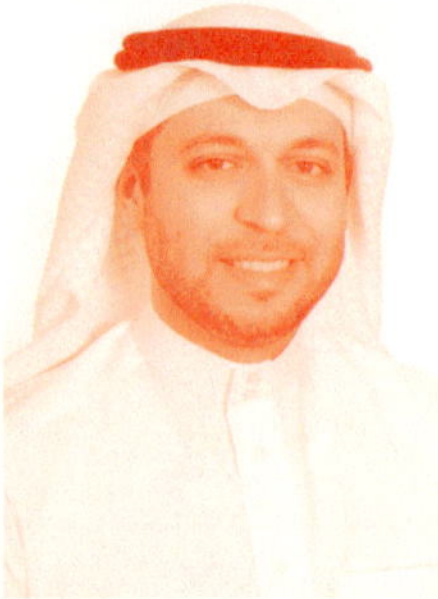
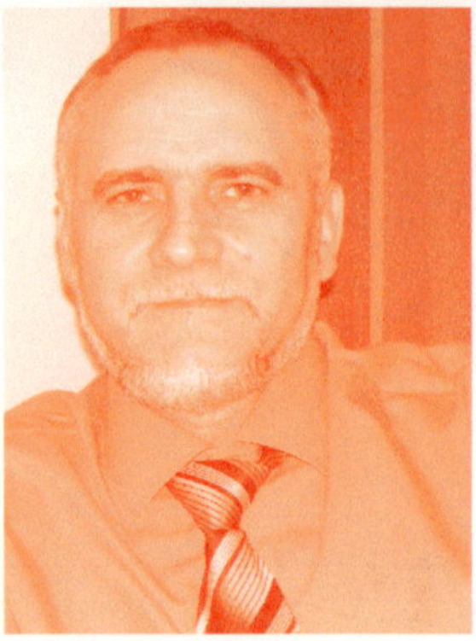
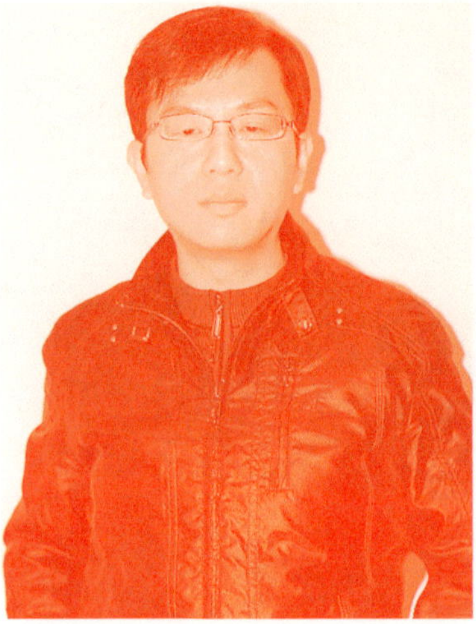
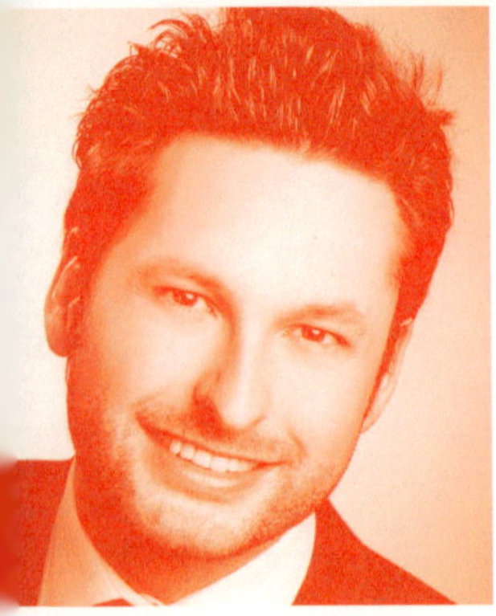
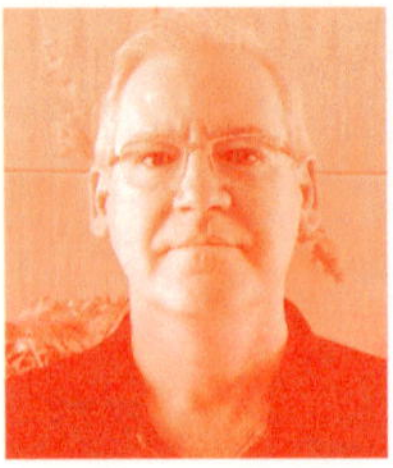

IntechOpen

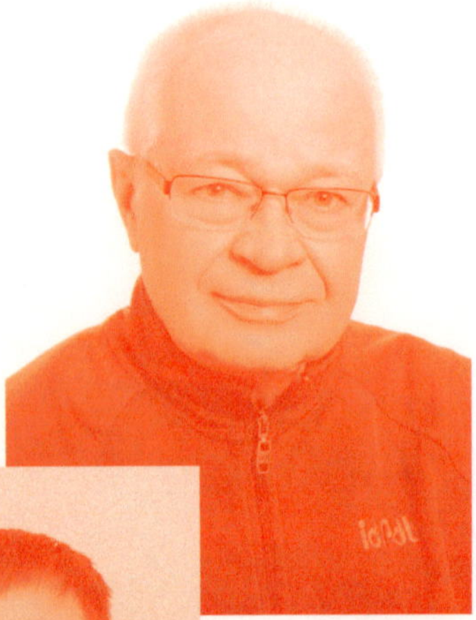
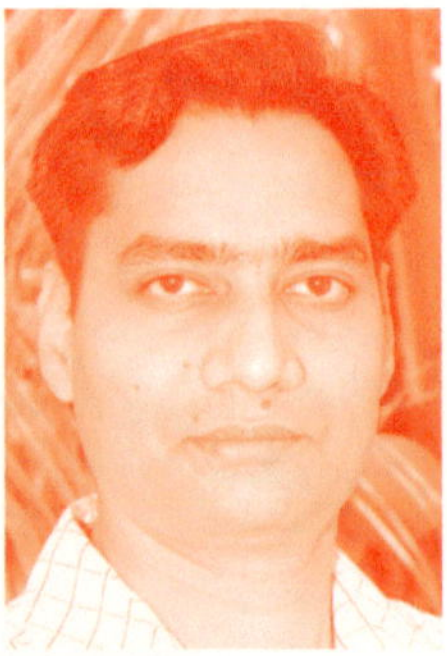
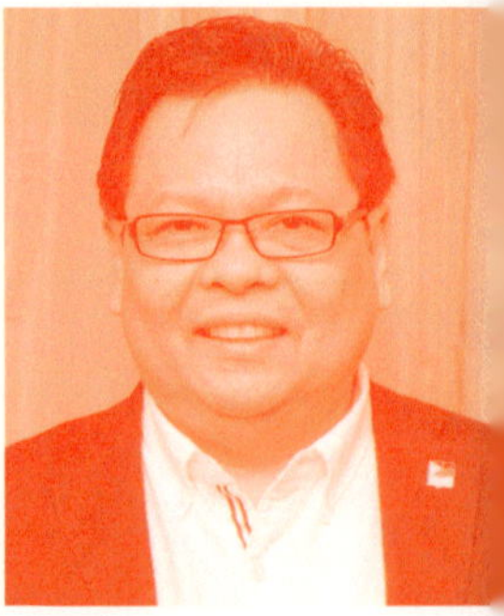
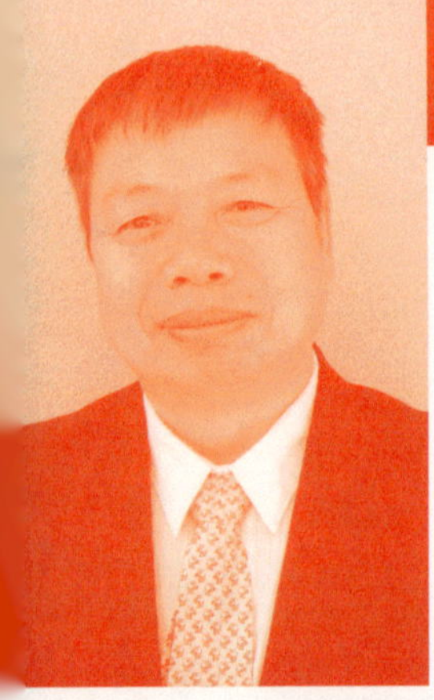
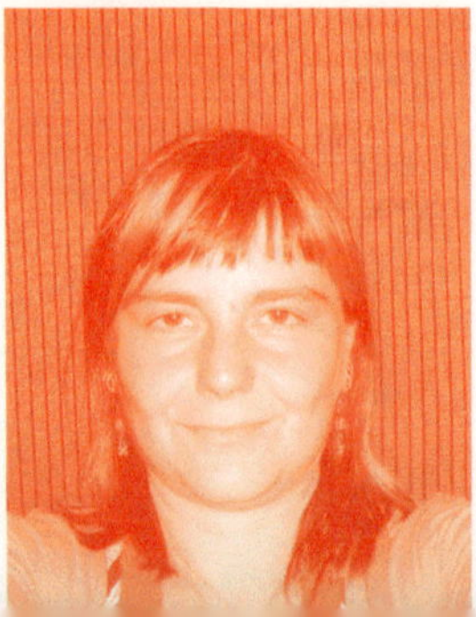
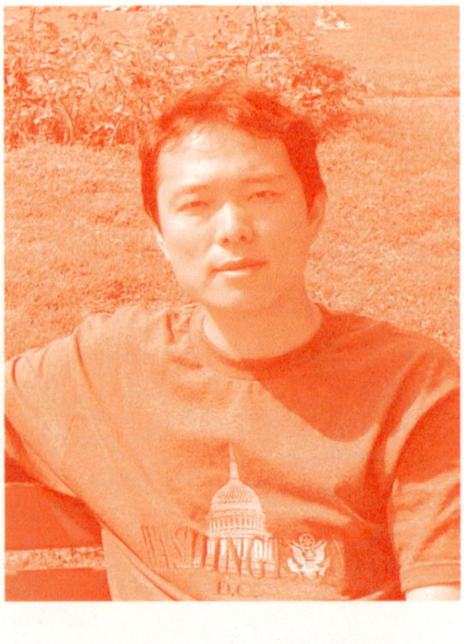

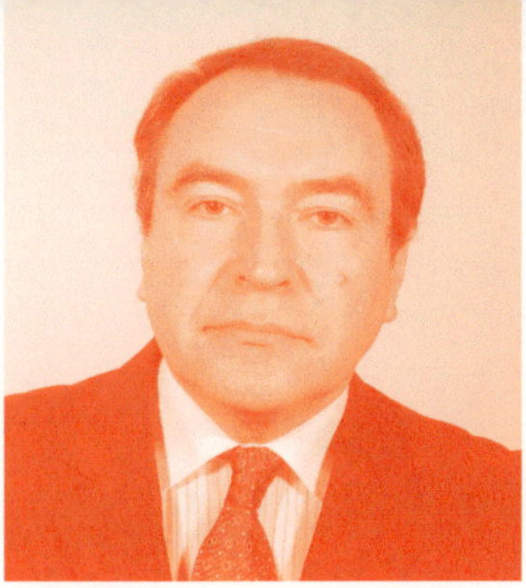
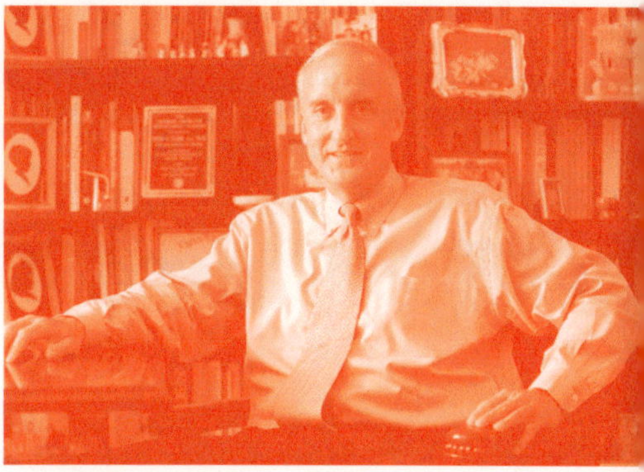
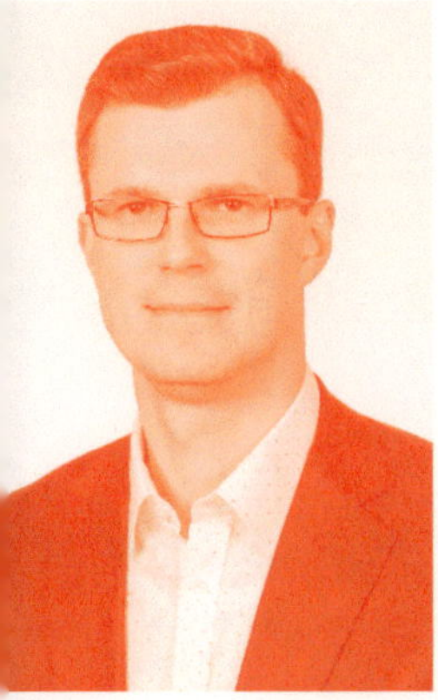
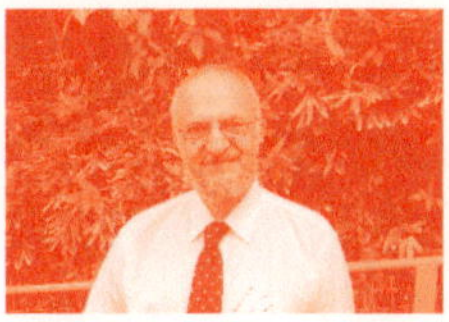
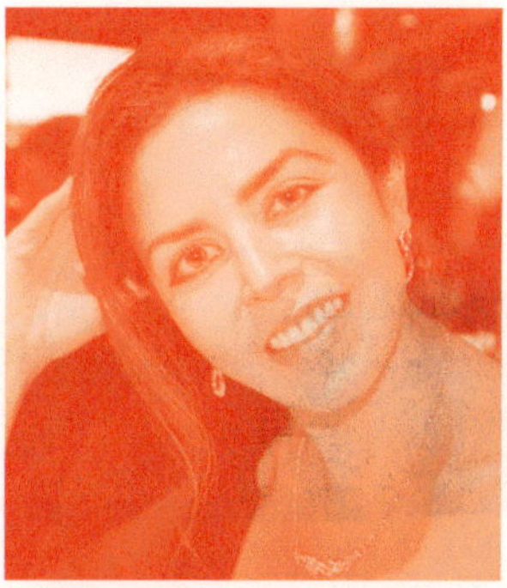

Supporting open minds since 2005

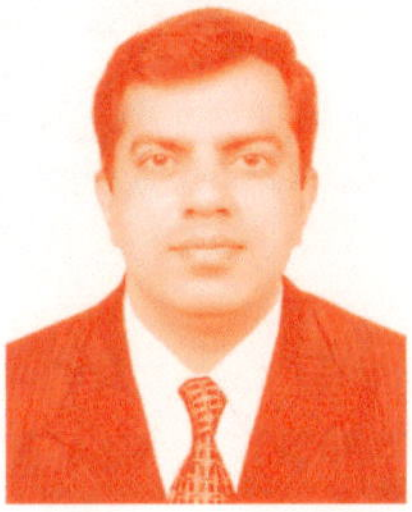
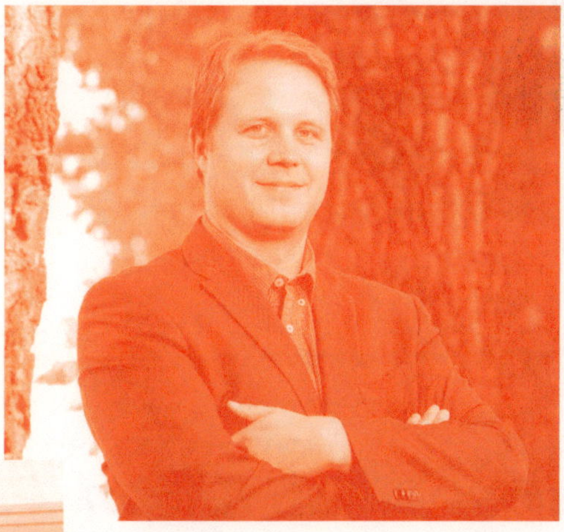
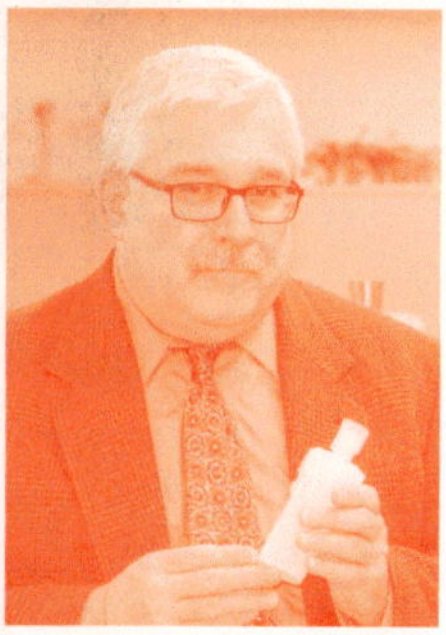
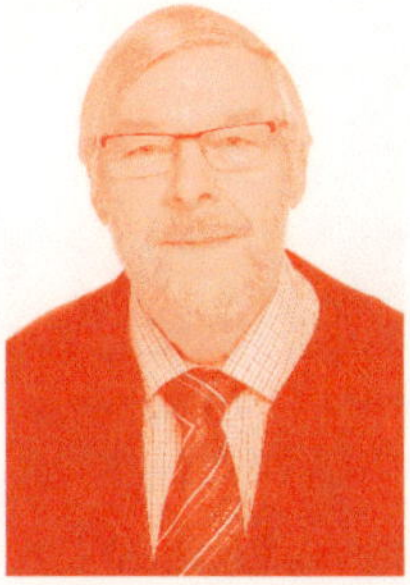
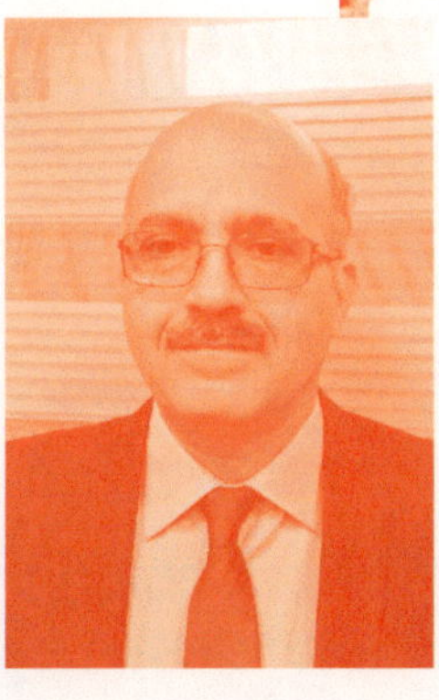
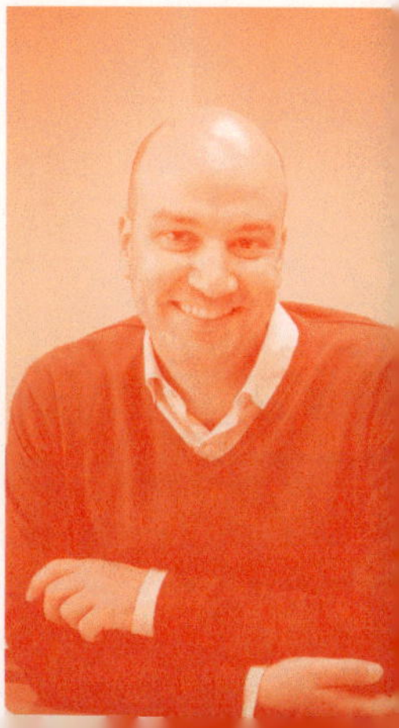
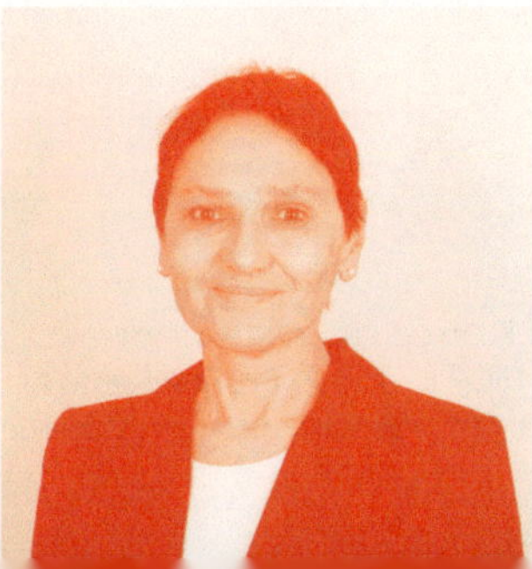

Human Papillomavirus
http://dx.doi.org/10.5772/intechopen.82907
Edited by Rajamanickam Rajkumar

Contributors
Vilas Nasare, Sanchita Roy Pradhan, Sutapa Mahata, Dipanwita Ghosh, Pranab Kumar Sahoo, Sinjini Sarkar, Ranita Pal, M. Faruk Kose, Emine Karabuk, Şerban Vifor Gabriel Berteşteanu, Raluca Grigore, Alexandru Nicolaescu, Mihnea Cojocarita-Condeescu, Suchibrata Das, Larisa Belotserkovtseva, Julia Mayer, Rajamanickam Rajkumar

First published in London, United Kingdom, 2020 by IntechOpen
IntechOpen is the global imprint of INTECHOPEN LIMITED, registered in England and Wales, registration number: 11086078, 7th floor, 10 Lower Thames Street, London, EC3R 6AF, United Kingdom
Printed in Croatia

British Library Cataloguing-in-Publication Data
A catalogue record for this book is available from the British Library

Additional hard and PDF copies can be obtained from orders@intechopen.com

Human Papillomavirus
Edited by Rajamanickam Rajkumar
p. cm.
Print ISBN 978-1-83881-219-5
Online ISBN 978-1-83881-220-1
eBook (PDF) ISBN 978-1-83881-221-8

For EU product safety concerns:
IN TECH d.o.o., Prolaz Marije Krucifikse Kozulić 3, 51000 Rijeka, Croatia, info@intechopen.com or visit our website at intechopen.com.

Meet the editor

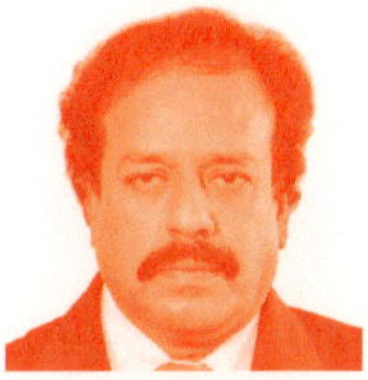

Rajamanickam Rajkumar is a scientists on the front lines of cervical cancer and HPV prevention and control. He has an MD in Community Medicine and a PhD in Cancer Epidemiology. He is currently a professor at Meenakshi Medical College Kanchipuram, India, and a PhD mentor at many medical universities. He was the principal investigator for one of the largest cervical cancer screening programs in India with technical support from the International Agency for Research on Cancer (IARC), a specialized agency of the World Health Organization. He conducted the first study in South India on the community prevalence of HPV. He has been trained in colposcopy and cancer epidemiology in France, Ireland, the United Kingdom, and Singapore. He is a consultant to the Ohio State University Medical University in Cervical Cancer Screening and an honorary member of the Society for Colposcopy & Cervical Pathology of Singapore (SCCPS). Since the start of 2020, he has served as Associate Research Director and Member Secretary of the Institutional Ethics Committee of Meenakshi Medical College. Dr. Rajkumar has won several awards, including Best Teacher and Researcher from the Meenakshi Academy of Higher Education and Research, India, in 2013, and Excellence in Research from the Institute of Scholars, India, in 2019.

Contents

Preface

In order to effectively contain and combat a virus, one has to understand the natural history of the virus and its microbiology, pathology, immunology, pathogenicity, clinical features, treatment and prevention options, and control measures. Never has this been clearer than now when the world is experiencing the COVID-19 pandemic. Of course, there are other viruses that must be dealt with as well.

This book is about the highly infective Human papillomavirus (HPV). There are more than 200 strains of HPV, though only a few, like HPV 16 and HPV 18, are oncogenic. HPV infections can lead to cancers of the cervix, vulva, vagina, anus, penis, and oral cavity.

Written by authors from across the globe, this book is a comprehensive look at HPV. Chapters cover such topics as the epidemiology of HPV, treatment of the manifestations of HPV, which can include warts on the skin and genitals, diagnosis and management of oral mucosal cancers due to HPV, HPV and pregnancy, and HPV vaccines.

This book serves as a useful reference for researchers and scientists, guiding them in the objective of eliminating HPV infections and related cancers, especially in developing countries with limited resources.

I am grateful to Dr. Rijula Raj, MPT, SRMIST, Chennai, Er. Rixon Raj, ME, MIT, Chennai, and Er. Pavith Raj for their valuable technical inputs. I thank my family Celin Rani and the lovely angel Helena Raj for their concern and care during the preparation of this book. My special thanks to Ms. Romina Rovan of IntechOpen publishing for her highly efficient management and skillful guidance during my editorship of this book.

Dr. Rajamanickam Rajkumar MD, PhD
Professor,
Community Medicine,
Meenakshi Medical College Hospital and Research Institute,
Meenakshi Academy of Higher Education and Research - MAHER,
Kanchipuram, Tamil Nadu, India

Chapter 1

The Importance of the Problem of HPV-Associated Diseases in KhMAO-Ugra: Vaccination of Adolescents against HPV - Problems and Prospects

Larisa Dmitrievna Belotserkovtseva and Yulia Igorevna Mayer

Abstract

In a survey of adolescents aged 14–17 years, we found that 25% already have experience of sexual contact and they do not know the methods of contraception and neglect condoms. About 77.6% of sexually active adolescent girls had genital infection, including HPV 52.7%, highly oncogenic types 37.9%, and mixed infections 51.4%. Adolescents are extremely vulnerable to HPV-related diseases. Cervical cancer takes the 2nd place in the structure of cancer in women in KHMAO-Ugra and the 1st place at the age of 30 years. Since 2009, girls have been vaccinated against HPV in Ugra. Over 10 years, there was a 39% decrease in the incidence of anogenital warts. We meet with parents, provide information about the risks of HPV infection, expose myths, and discuss the safety and effectiveness of HPV vaccines. Our goal is to win the trust of parents in vaccines, resist anti-vaccine propaganda, increase motivation, and reduce the number of refusal.

Keywords: papillomavirus, vaccination, cervical cancer, anogenital warts, adolescent reproductive behavior

1. The problem of HPV in Russia and in the Khanty-Mansiysk autonomous region-Ugra

Human papillomavirus (HPV) is the most frequent sexually transmitted infection. The prevalence of HPV in the world is about 10%.

HPV is the cause of a wide range of serious diseases in both men and women, including cancer and precancerous lesions of the cervix, vulva and vagina, anogenital area and anal canal, penis, and oropharynx, and also plays a crucial etiological role in the development of anogenital warts in both sexes [1–4]. Anogenital (venereal) warts are the most common clinical manifestation of HPV infection. More than 90% of all cases of anogenital warts are caused by 6 and 11 types of HPV. These types of HPV are also responsible for the development of recurrent respiratory papillomatosis [1–3, 5].

The problem of HPV infections during pregnancy can lead to complications such as intrauterine and intrapartum infections of the fetus, increased frequency of cesarean sections, and the risk of developing laryngeal papillomatosis of the larynx of the newborn, increasing the risk of infant mortality and the number of surgical interventions on the cervix for severe dysplasia in young women with risk of complications for subsequent pregnancies—spontaneous abortions and premature births.

2. Epidemiology of HPV-associated pathology in Russia and KhMAO-Ugra

Every year, more than 600,000 new cases of HPV-associated cancer are registered in the world, approximately 90% of which is cervical cancer. According to the statistics of the Russian Center for Information Technology and Epidemiological Research in Oncology of the Herzen Institute (branch of the Federal State Institute "National Medical Research Center of Radiology" of the Ministry of Health of the Russian Federation), in the structure of the incidence of malignant neoplasms of the population of the Russian Federation in 2015, cancers associated with HPV infection accounted for about 10% of the total incidence of cancer, and their total number was about 32,000 cases [6].

In the structure of female cancer incidence, cancers of the anogenital region are presented in different ways. Thus, cervical cancer in the Russian Federation occupies the 5th place (5.2%); cancer of the rectum, rectosigmoid junction, and anus, 6th place (4.6%); vulvar cancer, 20th place (0.6%); pharyngeal cancer (0.2%) and vaginal cancer (0.2%), 25–26th place; and laryngeal cancer—28th place (0.1%) [6].

However, if we consider the structure of oncological diseases of the female reproductive system, cervical cancer takes the second place in prevalence among malignant neoplasms of women under 45 years and the first in the number of lost years of life (the life expectancy of sick women is reduced by 26 years on average). The incidence of cervical cancer is steadily increasing and has increased by 28% on average over the past 10 years [7].

Only in 10 years, the incidence of cervical cancer in Russia has increased by an order of magnitude: from 7.9 per 100,000 of the female population in 2002 to 17.2—in 2012 [7]. In 2018, 17,000 new cases of cervical cancer and 6.6 thousand deaths were registered in the Russian Federation. In 2018, the incidence rate fell slightly to 15.76. Important markers characterizing the neglect of cervical cancer and the quality of treatment are the proportion of patients with advanced tumor process (3–4 stages), as well as the mortality of patients within a year from the moment of diagnosis, which in the Russian Federation in 2018 remained at a fairly high level: 34.6 and 13.8%, respectively. In the structure of disability, 83% of cases in oncogynecology are cervical cancer [8]. The frequent incidence of cervical cancer, the tendency to rejuvenate this pathology, a high percentage of neglected cases, and, as a consequence, the growth of disability among women of working age are a world problem, involving the most active, socially significant part of the female population. The occurrence of cervical cancer in young women is a serious social problem, causing deterioration in health, disability, and reduced fertility.

As for cancers of other localizations, annually in the Russian Federation, about 4000 cases of laryngeal cancer and 3000 deaths, for this reason, are registered. Morbidity and mortality from cancer of the vulva, vagina, anus, and penis in the Russian Federation are not registered, which is obviously due to low diagnosis and underreporting of cases. There are about 100,000 new cases of cancer of these locations in the world every year, and two-thirds of the incidence falls on women [8].

Anogenital (venereal) warts are the most common clinical manifestation of HPV infection, more than 90% of which are caused by HPV types 6 and 11. In Russia, this pathology is among the five leaders among sexually transmitted infections. It should be emphasized that the level of official registration is significantly different from the true prevalence and the possible true figure of the prevalence of anogenital warts, according to ongoing studies to assess the prevalence, can be more than 1,000,000 cases, which will bring this nosology to the first place in frequency among all recorded genital infections. The lack of specific antiviral therapy, as well as frequent relapses after the use of destructive methods, complicates the treatment of the disease, significantly reducing the quality of life of these patients [9].

The average annual population of Khanty-Mansiysk Autonomous Region-Ugra is 1,659,436 people, of which 851,588 are women and 805,848 are men.

Cervical cancer in our region occupies the second place in the structure of tumors of the reproductive system of women and the first place in the age category up to 30 years. Precancerous lesions of the cervix are detected more than 6000 cases per year [10].

The clinical burden of cancer (cervical cancer, vulvar and vaginal cancer, anal cancer) among the female population in our region is up to 300 cases per year, which is relevant within the workload of cancer beds and rationalization of health-care costs. In KhMAO-Ugra, according to the state registration, the incidence of cervical cancer does not tend to decrease: in 2018, it was 14.7 per 100 thousand population and in Russia 15.76. The number of registered women diagnosed with cervical cancer is steadily increasing. Annually in Ugra, about 160–170 cases of cervical cancer are registered for the first time. Among the newly identified cases, every second patient (50.8%) is under the reproductive age of 45 years and every third woman (33.2%) had an advanced stage 3–4 of the disease. About 12–15% of patients with cervical cancer die in the first year of diagnosis. Mortality from this disease in Ugra in 2018 was 6.0 per 100,000 population; in 2018 54 women died [10].

The standard screening procedure in KhMAO-Ugra, as well as in the world, is the PAP test, the effectiveness of which does not exceed 30–40%. Despite the introduction of modern methods and some progress in diagnosis and treatment, cancer prevention is still crucial.

3. Study of the expression of oncoprotein E7 in the diagnosis of cervical diseases associated with human papillomavirus

Infection caused by human papillomavirus occurs in 50–80% of the population and in 99.7% of cases of confirmed cervical cancer and therefore is an important problem of modern health care. First of all, this applies to the pathology of the cervix, which is the most important organ of the reproductive system of a woman. Thus, recent data indicate a fourfold increase in cases of cervical cancer among women under 35 years. The incidence of papillomavirus infection in general has also increased, which occurs in 44% of women who have seen a gynecologist. Against the background of persistent HPV of the urogenital tract, most cervical intraepithelial neoplasms develop, which in 15–20% of cases can end in oncological pathology (carcinoma in situ and invasive cancer) [3, 6, 9].

Given the high prevalence of papillomavirus infection, the uncertainty of its outcome, it is important to determine the phase of interaction of HPV with the cell. During the reproduction of HPV in the body, there is a persistence of its genome in the episomal form with the production of viral particles. In this phase of reproduction, there is a high probability of spontaneous remission [2, 9].

The integrative phase is characterized by the embedding of HPV DNA sequences of the 16th and 18th serotypes into the chromosome of the infected cell, which is accompanied by the synthesis of oncoprotein E7. Viral particles are not produced. Expression of oncoprotein E7 is a factor that significantly increases the risk of oncogenic transformation of the cervical epithelium. Increased synthesis of oncoprotein E7, a product of the viral genome, indicates an integrative phase of HPV-cell interaction in which the probability of spontaneous remission is low. However, this pattern is not absolute, as some cases in malignant tumors identified episomal form of HPV DNA or a combination of episomal and integrated forms [11, 12].

The insufficient number of clinical studies on the content of oncoprotein E7 in HPV does not yet allow for widespread use of this indicator in practical health care.

The aim of the study was to study the level of expression of cancer protein E7 in patients with cervical pathology with positive and negative HPV tests [11, 12].

Materials and methods: We conducted a continuous randomized prospective study. According to the results of HPV testing by polymerase chain reaction (PCR), all patients with cervical pathology (95 women) were divided into two groups: the 1 group (control group) (HPV-negative, n = 57) and the 2 group (main group)(HPV-positive, n = 38). Group 1 (control group), consisting of 57 women with cervical pathology (HPV-negative test) was divided into two subgroups by analysis for the presence of oncoprotein E7 expression. In first subgroup, 13 women had a positive result which is 1 E7-positive subgroup, and 44 women had a negative result which is 1 E7-negative subgroup. Group 2 (main group) consisting of 38 women with cervical pathology, were infected with human papillomavirus of high carcinogenic risk. Group 2 (main group) was divided into two subgroups: subgroup of 11 women is 2 E7-positive subgroup, who tested positive for oncoprotein E7, and of 27 women, whose E7 was not detected—a negative result is 2 E7-negative subgroup.

Clinical observation and bacteriological, bacterioscopic, cytological, endoscopic (colposcopy), and histomorphological methods were used during the examination. All women were tested for papillomavirus infection. Verification of the diagnosis of papillomavirus infection was carried out by polymerase chain reaction. Quantitative determination of oncoprotein E7 in cervical samples was carried out using the enzyme immunoassay system NPF "Mirax-Pharma" (Moscow). Purified recombinant type 16 protein E7 was titrated as standard. The optical density, which is critical for each formulation, was determined. The test result of the sample was considered positive if the optical density was greater than or equal to the critical. The result of the sample study was considered negative if the optical density was less than the critical one. A survey card was filled in for each patient.

The comparison was carried out on the basis of sample averages (M), medians (Me), and standard deviation (Q25–Q75). Statistical analysis was performed using the nonparametric Mann–Whitney criterion (U) for independent groups. The reliability of the differences between the percentages of the two samples was estimated by the value of the Fisher angular distribution criterion (φ). The values at $p < 0.05$ were considered reliable.

4. Results and discussion

The average age of the patients, the onset of menstrual function, the duration of their residence in the North, and the onset of sexual life were comparable in all groups and had no statistical significance ($p > 0.05$). The number of sexual partners had statistical significance in 1 E7-negative subgroup of the control group compared with the main group—2.00 (2.00–3.00), 2.00 (1.00–3.00), 3.00 (2.00–7.00), and

3.00 (2.00–5.00), respectively (2–3,4*p < 0.05). In the study of obstetric history, the number of births and abortions in all groups had no statistical significance (p > 0.05).

In the study of somatic history in 2 E7-positive subgroup, kidney disease accounted for 27.3% and endocrine disease 27.3% and had statistical significance in comparison with 1 E7-negative subgroup (*p < 0.05), respectively.

In the study of hereditary oncological history, oncological diseases were found in relatives, 15.38, 40.91, 45.45, and 22.22% in subgroups, respectively (21–2, 3*p < 0.05; 2–4*p < 0.05), where in the 2 E7-positive subgroup, a burdened family oncological history was revealed in 45.45% of cases.

In the study of gynecological history, we paid attention to diseases that could serve as additional factors in the development of neoplasia and cervical cancer. Among gynecological pathology, inflammatory diseases of the female genital organs in the 2 E7-positive subgroup were significantly more common, such as endometritis (27.27%) (3–2*p < 0.05), vulvovaginitis (90.90%) (*p < 0.05), and salpingo-oophoritis (36.36%) (3–4*p < 0.05); inflammatory diseases can reduce immunity and stimulate the tumor process. Infection of the genitourinary organs by pathogens of sexually transmissible infections according to the anamnesis also prevailed in the 2 E7-positive subgroup, such as *Ureaplasma* (27.27%), *Mycoplasma* (18.18%), and *Chlamydia* infection (18.18%) (4–2*p < 0.05), which required an in-depth study of the anamnesis and examination of the sexual partner.

Attention is drawn to a large number of cervical pathology in history. Cervical diseases in the history of patients in subgroups had, respectively, 84.62, 88.64, 100.00, and 81.42%.

When cytological examination of patients for atypical cells is performed, signs of cervical intraepithelial neoplasia (CIN) were found in 45,5, 61,54, 77,3, 81,81, and 66.66% (1–3* * p < 0.01; 1–4. 5*p < 0.05) in subgroups, respectively (**Table 1**).

A HPV effect was observed in patients only in 1 E7-negative (in 4.5% of cases) and 2 E7-positive (in 18.2% of cases); the reliability was confirmed in comparison with the control group (3,4–1,2**p < 0.01).

In recent years, the impact of sexually transmitted infections on the likelihood of developing dysplasia and cervical cancer has been considered. The structure of chronic inflammatory diseases of the cervical canal and cervix is currently dominated by cervicitis caused by *Chlamydia trachomatis* in combination with human papillomavirus. In these conditions, CIN and possibly cervical cancer often develop. Many researchers note that *Chlamydia* infection is a cofactor in the occurrence of cervical intraepithelial neoplasia in the presence of HPV.

Chlamydia infection was found only in 2 E7-positive subgroup (9.1%); *Ureaplasma* infection also prevailed in this subgroup (27.3%) (3–2*p < 0.05). *Mycoplasma* infection prevailed in the 2 E7-positive subgroup (14.8%) (4–1**p < 0.01) (**Table 2**).

Group mark	Control group HPV (−)		Main group HPV (+)	
	1 E7-positive (n = 13)[1]	1 E7-negative (n = 44)[2]	2 E7-positive (n = 11)[3]	2 E7-negative (n = 27)[4]
NILM	38,46% (5)	25,00% (11)	18,18% (2)	33,33% (9)
LSIL	61,54% (8)	77,27% (34)	81,81% (9)	66,66% (18)
HSIL	7,69% (1)	4,54% (2)	18,18% (2)	14,81% (4)
HPV effect	0,00% (0)*3	2,27% (1)*3	18,18% (2)**4	0,00% (0)

*φ **p < 0,01; φ *p < 0,05.*

Table 1.
The results of the PAP test.

Infection with human papillomavirus in women with cervical pathology was confirmed in 40% of patients. In the main group, a positive test for HPV type 16 was detected in 68.4% (26 women) and HPV type 18 in 42.1% (16 women). The combination of HPV 16 and 18 genotypes was found in 10.5% (4 women). HPV type 16 infection in the main group was found in subgroups 54.54 and 74.07%, respectively, and HPV type 18 was found in subgroups 54.54 and 37.04%, respectively.

Thus, HPV infection alone is not enough to induce tumor growth and confirms the role of mixed infection as a cofactor in HPV-dependent carcinogenesis.

During colposcopy (**Table 3**), the condition of the cervix and vagina was assessed, the localization and boundaries of the lesion were determined, benign changes were differentiated from suspected malignancies, and cytological smears and biopsies were taken from suspicious areas of the cervix. Among the results of a colposcopic view, 2 E7-positive and 2 E7-negative subgroups prevailed of CIN (45.45%) (3-2* $p < 0.05$). Atypical vessels were determined in 63.63% (3–2** $p < 0.01$; 3–1*$p < 0.05$) and 59.26% (4–2**$p < 0.01$; 4–1*$p < 0.05$), respectively; the mosaic in the subgroups was 54.54% (3–2** $p < 0.01$; 3–1*$p < 0.05$) and 44.44% (4–2**$p < 0.01$; 4–1*$p < 0.05$), respectively.

In the group of HPV-positive women, abnormal colposcopic views (iodine-negative epithelium, punctuation, mosaic, aceto-white epithelium, atypical vessels) were much more common, which confirms the damaging effect of the human

Group mark	**Control group HPV (−)**		**Main group HPV (+)**	
	1 E7-positive (n = 13)^{1}	**1 E7-negative (n = 44)^{2}**	**2 E7-positive (n = 11)^{3}**	**2 E7-negative (n = 27)^{4}**
Chlamydia trachomatis	0,00% (0)	0,00% (0)^{*3}	9,09% (1)^{*4}	0,00% (0)
Ureaplasma spp.	15,38% (2)	6,82% (3)^{*3}	27,27% (3)	11,11% (3)
Mycoplasma spp.	0,00% (0)^{*2**4}	9,09% (4)	9,09% (1)	14,81% (4)
HPV 16	0,00% (0)^{**3,4}	0,00% (0)^{**3,4}	54,54% (6)	74,07% (20)
HPV 18	0,00% (0)^{**3,4}	0,00% (0)^{**3,4}	54,54% (6)	37,04% (10)

φ $^{**}p < 0,01$; $^{*}p < 0,05$; φ $^{*}p < 0,05$.

Table 2.
Results of examination for sexually transmitted infections.

Group mark	**Control group HPV (−)**		**Main group HPV (+)**	
	1 E7-positive (n = 13)^{1}	**1 E7-negative (n = 44)^{2}**	**2 E7-positive (n = 11)^{3}**	**2 E7-negative (n = 27)^{4}**
Normal	0,00% (0)	0,00% (0)	0,00% (0)	0,00% (0)
Aceto-white epithelium	23,08% (3)^{*4}	13,64% (6)^{*3**4}	45,45% (5)	55,55% (15)
CIS	0,00% (0)	0,00% (0)^{*3}	9,09% (1)	3,70% (1)
Atypical vessels	23,08% (3)^{*3,4}	18,18% (8)^{**3,4}	63,63% (7)	59,26% (16)
Mosaic	15,38% (2)^{*3,4}	11,36% (5)^{**3,4}	54,54% (6)	44,44% (12)
Punctuation	0,00% (0)	4,54% (2)	9,09% (1)	7,40% (2)

φ $^{**}p < 0,01$; $^{*}p < 0,05$; φ $^{*}p < 0,05$.

Table 3.
Extended colposcopy results.

papillomavirus on the state of the cervical epithelium and complicates the course of pathological processes toward carcinogenesis. All abnormal colposcopic views were indications for biopsy. Tissue for biopsy was taken by radio-wave loop.

Histological examination revealed the following results (**Table 4**). Signs of chronic inflammatory process prevailed in the control group and amounted to 61.54% and 56.82%, respectively (2–1, 3–1* * p < 0.01). Signs of stationary endocervicosis were found in the control group (30.77 and 38.63%, respectively) and in the main group (18.18 and 33.33%, respectively). This had no statistical significance (p > 0.05). Epidermizing endocervicosis prevailed in 2 E7-positive, and its detection rate was 45.45% (4–1* * p < 0.01; 4–5*p < 0.05).

CIN I, II, and III prevailed in women with HPV (+) in the main group, and according to the results of histological conclusion, CIN I was found in subgroup 2 E7-positive in 36.36% of cases (4–1* * p < 0.01; 4–2*p < 0.05) and in subgroup 2 E7-negative in 40.74% of cases (5–1,2**p < 0.01).

CIN II was diagnosed in the main group in 27.27% (4-1**p < 0.01) and in 29.63% of cases (5-1**p < 0.01; 5-3*p < 0.05), respectively, subgroups. CIN III was observed in women with HPV (+) of the main group in 27.27% (4–1,3**p < 0.01) and in 22.22% of cases (4–1,3**p < 0.01), respectively. Cancer in situ was diagnosed in the main group in 9.09% (4-3*p < 0.05) and 7.40% of cases (5-1,3*p < 0.05), respectively, subgroups, indicating the role of HPV in the carcinogenesis of cervical cancer.

Signs of koilocytosis were determined in subgroups 0, 7,69, 2,27, 54,54, and 51.85%, respectively. In women with HPV (+) of the main group, these indicators were maximum and had statistical significance (4,5–1,2,3**p < 0.01). It should be noted that the maximum of abnormal colposcopic species were women in subgroups with increased expression of oncoprotein E7.

Thus, in the group of HPV-positive women, according to the results of histological examination, cervical intraepithelial neoplasia of medium and severe degree and cervical cancer were more common. Moreover, koilocytic transformation of the epithelium, CIN III, and cervical cancer was diagnosed more often in subgroup

Group mark	Control group HPV (−)		Main group HPV (+)	
	1 E7-positive (n = 13)¹	**1 E7-negative (n = 44)²**	**2 E7-positive (n = 11)³**	**2 E7-negative (n = 27)⁴**
No evidence	0,00% (0)	0,00% (0)	0,00% (0)	0,00% (0)
Chronic cervicitis	61,54% (8)	56,82% (25)	45,45% (5)	55,55% (15)
Stationary endocervicosis	30,77% (4)	38,63% (17)	18,18% (2)	33,33% (9)
Epidermizing endocervicosis	38,46% (5)	38,63% (17)*4	45,45% (5)*4	18,52% (5)
Leukoplakia	23,08% (3)	9,09% (4)	18,18% (2)	18,52% (5)
CIN I	7,69% (1)*3**4	22,72% (10)	36,36%(4)	40,74%(11)
CIN II	15,38% (2)	9,09% (4)*4	27,27% (3)	29,63% (8)
CIN III	7,69% (1)*2	0,00% (0)**3,4	27,27% (3)	22,22% (6)
Cervical cancer	0,00% (0)	0,00% (0)*4	9,09% (1)	7,40% (2)
Koilocytes	7,69% (1)**3,4	2,27% (1)**3,4	54,54% (6)	51,85% (14)

***p < 0,01; *p < 0,05.*

Table 4.
Results of histological examination.

2 E7-positive than in subgroup 2 E7-negative, according to the conclusion of morphologists.

The results of the study of the level of expression of cancer protein E7 are presented in **Table 5**. Indicators were distributed according to subgroups: 0,087 (0,07–0,12); 0,190 (0,18–0,39); 0,074 (0,06–0,10); 0,200 (0,17–0,31); and 0.081 (0.07–0.10) (**p < 0.01). We found a significant increase in the indicator in the main group (2 E7-positive), compared with the control group 1 E7-negative and 2 E7-negative (**p < 0.01). In the main group (subgroup 1 E7-positive), this indicator also had statistical significance in comparison with subgroups 1 E7-negative and 2 E7-negative (**p < 0.01).

The increased expression of oncoprotein E7 in the main group (2 E7-positive) was maximal in comparison with subgroups 1 E7-negative and 2 E7-negative (**p < 0.01), which is an indicator of the aggressiveness of the incipient tumor process and a criterion for an unfavorable prognosis. In subgroup 1 E7-positive, increased expression of oncoprotein E7 was also detected in comparison with the control 1 E7-negative subgroup and the main 2 E7-negative subgroup (**p < 0.01).

As a result of studying the level of expression of oncoprotein E7 in HPV-positive and HPV-negative women, we made the following conclusions:

1. In the group of women with cervical pathology associated with human papillomavirus infection, an increased frequency of abnormal colposcopic views, mosaic (3.5 times higher, p <0.01), acetone-white epithelium (2.4 times higher, p < 0.05), atypical vessels (3.5 times higher, p <0.01), punctuation (2.3 times more often, p <0.05), as well as cytological examination, LSIL signs (2.4 times higher), HSIL was found only in the HPV group (p <0.01), and histological examination of CIN I found is 4.7 times higher (p < 0.05), CIN II is 3.2 times more likely (p < 0.05), CIN III is 22.3 times more often (p < 0.01), and cervical cancer is 7.89%. This confirms the damaging effect of the human papillomavirus on the cervical epithelium and complicates the course of pathological processes toward carcinogenesis.

2. The results of the study showed that in cervical pathology caused by HPV of high carcinogenic risk, the increased content of cancer protein E7 is detected 2.5 times (p < 0.01) more often than in women that are HPV (−). The level of E7 indicates an aggressive process of carcinogenesis and can be considered as an unfavorable prognostic sign.

Group mark	Control group HPV (−)		Main group HPV (+)		Statistic parameters
	1 E7-positive (n = 13)[1]	1 E7-negative (n = 44)[2]	1 E7-positive (n = 13)[1]	1 E7-negative (n = 44)[2]	Kruskall-Wallis
	Me (Q_{25}–Q_{75})	Me (Q_{25}–Q_{75})	Me (Q_{25}–Q_{75})	Me (Q_{25}–Q_{75})	χ^2
E7	0,190 (0,18–0,39) U**2,4	0,074 (0,06–0,10) U**2,4	0,200 (0,17–0,31) U**4	0,081 (0,07–0,10)	33,116 p < 0,001
ОП крит	0,145 (0,145–0,196)	0,145 (0,145–0,196)	0,145 (0,145–0,196)	0,145 (0,145–0,196)	

*Kruskall-Wallis: χ2; p (**p < 0,01; *p < 0,05); Mann–Whitney (U) U **p < 0.*

Table 5.
The results of the study of the level of expression of the oncoprotein E7.

3. Laboratory test evaluation of oncogenic transformation of the cervical epithelium requires further study, as it allows in conjunction with other diagnostic methods to determine the group of increased oncogenic risk among patients with gynecological diseases. The proven relationship between elevated levels of expression of oncoprotein E7 and the presence of CIN allows us to recommend the definition of oncoprotein E7 for inclusion in the diagnostic program for HPV-positive women with changes in the cervix and pathological cervical smears.

5. Teenagers are a risk group: reproductive behavior and adolescent reproductive health

Biological susceptibility to HPV and structural immaturity of the cervix in adolescence, high frequency of ectopia of the cylindrical epithelium, and activation of squamous metaplasia processes create optimal conditions for the introduction and replication of human papillomavirus, which makes the adolescent population extremely vulnerable to the development of CIN.

Features of reproductive behavior of adolescents determine the risks that contribute to the development of diseases of the reproductive system. These are the early beginning of sexual life, frequent change of sexual partners due to the absence of persistent lasting relations in paired unlike adults, who create families and in most adhere to monogamous relations. As a result of adolescents' neglect of barrier contraception, they have a high incidence of sexually transmitted infections. Early sexual life and especially sexual behavior of adolescents contribute to the spread of sexual infections among them, which often remain undiagnosed and not treated in time [13].

Physiological features of the anatomy of the cervix in adolescent girls' anatomy create prerequisites for the persistence of HPV in the epithelial cells of the cervix of the girl; long-term persistence of the virus can lead to the development of precancerous lesions and cervical cancer. *Chlamydia* and *Mycoplasma* infections associated with HPV are cofactors that exacerbate the situation. Age-related physiological ectopia of the cylindrical epithelium, characteristic of adolescence, and defective hormonal homeostasis lead to a violation of the physiological barriers of the genitals. The cylindrical epithelium is an ideal environment for papillomavirus invasion due to the availability of reserve cells and the large area of the transformation zone [14].

Promiscuity and unsettled partnerships are of primary importance in early HPV infection and increased risk of CIN against the background of high infection rates among adolescents with sexually transmitted infections.

In sexually active girls, genital inflammation is detected three times more often (45.2%) than in their peers who do not live a sexual life—in 15.1% of girls. Pathology of the cervix at the age of 18 is detected in 33.4% of girls. According to the results of the survey of sexually active adolescents for genital infections, sexually transmissible infections were detected in 77.8%, including *Mycoplasma genitalium*, 18.4%; *Chlamydia trachomatis*, 6.2%; and HPV, 52.7% (including highly oncogenic types—34.7%), and mixed infections in 51.4%. In KhMAO-Ugra, the HPV infection rate of girls aged 14–16 is 40%, and among girls aged 17–18, the infection rate increases to 60% [13].

We conducted an anonymous survey of schoolchildren in Surgut, which was attended by 389 high school students, including 201 girls and 188 boys aged from 14 to 18. The median age was 16.9 years. Among them, 24% have experience of sexual contact. About 50% of sexually active adolescents indicated that they had a sexual debut at the age of 16 and younger. About 14.6% of them had the first sexual contact at the age of 15, 10.4% from 13 to 14 years old, 31.2% from 17 years old, and 16.7% from 18 years old. About 66.7% of them had 1 sexual partner; every third (33.3%) sexually active teenager under the age of 18 had 2 or more sexual partners. For contraception, 57% of respondents use a condom, 29%—combined oral contraceptives. Only 23.5% of adolescents are regularly protected from sexual infections, 27% never use barrier contraception.

6. Introduction of vaccination of adolescents against HPV infection in KhMAO-Ugra: problems and solutions

The strategic direction of the development of modern health care in the Russian Federation is prevention and early detection of diseases, which contributes to more effective treatment and improvement of demographic indicators of public health. One of the most important preventive measures is vaccination, and today more than 30 diseases that cause serious damage to human health can be prevented with its help. Immunization prevents 2.5 million deaths per year across all age groups.

These facts indicate that the issues of prevention and treatment of HPV-associated diseases require a multidisciplinary approach, as they affect such specialists as gynecologists, oncologists, epidemiologists, pediatricians, immunologists, dermatologists, etc.

The World Health Organization has been recommending the inclusion of HPV vaccination in vaccination calendars around the world since 2009 [15]. The WHO and the United Nations Children's Fund (UNICEF) consider HPV vaccination a priority for national immunization programs. More than 60 countries have already introduced universal mass vaccination of girls; in a number of countries (the USA, Australia, Canada, Austria, New Zealand, etc.), boys are vaccinated along with girls.

To date, the Russian Federation has two documents regulating measures for the prevention of HPV-associated diseases.

1. "Federal clinical guidelines for the management of patients with anogenital (venereal) warts," Russian society of dermatovenerologists and cosmetologists, (Moscow, 2015). For the prevention of diseases associated with HPV, two vaccines are registered in the Russian Federation: bivalent and quadrivalent. The bivalent HPV vaccine is used to prevent cancer and precancerous diseases of the cervix, vulva, and vagina in women aged 9 to 45 years. Quadrivalent HPV vaccine is used for the prevention of cancer and precancerous changes of the cervix; vulva cancer, vagina cancer, and anal cancer; and anogenital warts in women from 9 to 45 years, as well as anal cancer and anogenital warts in men from 9 to 26 years [16].

2. "Federal clinical guidelines for HPV vaccine prevention," Union of Pediatricians of Russia (Moscow, 2016). These clinical guidelines regulate two vaccination regimens. Standard scheme: girls/women from 14 to 45 years old and boys/men from 14 to 26 years old—three doses (0–2–6 months). Alternative scheme: girls and boys from 9 to 13 years old—it is possible to carry out two-dose immunization (0–6 months) [17].

Despite government HPV vaccination programs, female vaccination rates remain below targets in many countries [18, 19]. Models tend to demonstrate that vaccination of boys is most cost-effective if vaccination coverage of the female population is at a suboptimal level (less than 50%) [20, 21]. The benefits of vaccinating adolescent boys are not only the prevention of HPV infection for the partner but also the prevention of cancer of the penis and anal canal and anogenital warts.

Vaccination is the most effective investment in health care. The cost of treatment of one case of cervical cancer in the Russian Federation on average is $3000 and the cost of vaccination with preventive vaccination Gardasil—$235. With mass immunization of adolescents aged 12 years old, the pharmacoeconomic efficacy of vaccine introduction was calculated on a national scale, which showed the amount of prevented costs to be $235,000,000, and in the first 5 years, only $16,000,000 will be prevented by reducing genital warts [22].

There are numerous publications confirming the pharmacoeconomic effectiveness of HPV vaccination not only in computational models but also in real life [22–28].

In 2013, the Research Institute of Childhood Infections of the FMBA conducted a pharmacoeconomical evaluation of the cost-effectiveness of vaccination of 12-year-old girls with a quadrivalent HPV vaccine in Russia. For the period of survival, taking into account both direct medical and indirect costs, the vaccine is characterized by a cost-effectiveness ratio equal to $5800/QALY. When the gross domestic product of the Russian Federation was $6000, vaccination of girls with a quadrivalent HPV vaccine in the Russian Federation is characterized by high cost efficiency and can be recommended for routine use in the Russian population.

According to the instructions, the vaccine is approved for use in women aged 9 to 45 years old and in men aged 9 to 26 years old and can protect against diseases such as cervical cancer, vulvar cancer, vaginal cancer, anal cancer, and anogenital warts. Due to the fact that the human papillomavirus causes serious diseases in men, and screening methods for HPV-associated lesions of the anal canal and penis do not exist today, universal vaccination of adolescents of both sexes with quadrivalent HPV vaccine, the only one approved for use in boys, will achieve significant results in reducing the level of HPV-associated diseases and the rapid spread of HPV infection in the world [29].

The primary target cohort for HPV vaccination is children and adolescents aged 9 to 13 years before sexual debut, as recommended by the World Health Organization. The WHO since 2009 recommends that vaccination against human papillomavirus be included in vaccination calendars of all countries of the world. The WHO and the United Nations Children's Fund consider HPV vaccination as a priority for national immunization programs. Sixty countries have already introduced universal mass vaccination of girls, and three countries (the USA, Australia, Canada) also vaccinate boys against HPV.

At the moment, two HPV vaccines are registered in the Russian Federation: bivalent vaccine (Cervarix, contains antigens to 16 and 18 types of HPV) and quadrivalent vaccine (Gardasil, contains antigens 6, 11, 16, and 18 types of HPV). Bivalent HPV vaccine is used to prevent cancer and precancerous lesions of the cervix, vulva, and vagina. Quadrivalent HPV vaccine can protect not only from cervical, vulvar, and vaginal cancer but also from cancer of the anal canal and anogenital warts in women and men. The primary target cohort for HPV vaccination is adolescents aged 9–13 years old prior to sexual debut, as recommended by the World Health Organization [1].

The monitoring of epidemiological effectiveness is an integral part of HPV vaccination programs. In the long term, HPV vaccination can reduce the incidence and mortality from a number of cancers (cervical cancer, anal cancer, etc.), the prevention of which is a public health priority. Evaluation of the effectiveness of vaccination programs in the medium term is possible to reduce precancerous dysplasia and in the short term (2–4 years from the beginning of the program)—to reduce the prevalence of anogenital warts. Experience with national HPV vaccination programs has shown that maximum coverage can be achieved with school-based vaccination, as recommended by the WHO.

Since 2007, 27 regional programs of primary prevention of HPV-associated diseases have been implemented in Russia, which indicates the importance of protection against HPV infection.

A decrease in the incidence of anogenital warts in the general population has been recorded in the USA, Australia, New Zealand, Belgium, Sweden, and Germany. For example, in Australia, 4 years after the introduction of vaccination, there were the almost complete disappearance of anogenital warts in the population of young women and almost 40% reduction in precancerous lesions of the cervix in young women. The rate of decline was clearly correlated with vaccination coverage. The greatest effect was observed in countries with high coverage (70–85%) [26, 27, 30–33].

The experience of such regions as KhMAO, where the vaccination calendar is constantly being improved and the result is evaluated, can be an example for other regions and become one of the arguments for expanding the national calendar of preventive vaccinations.

The regional HPV vaccination program for adolescent girls in KHMAO was launched in 2009. In the process of introducing the vaccination program, we faced a number of difficulties and objections, which were mainly related to the lack of awareness of pediatricians and parents, and a lot of myths and negative reviews on the Internet and in the media.

We studied the opinions of parents and doctors on the vaccine prevention of HPV-associated diseases. Our goal was to raise awareness among parents and health-care providers and to assess the impact of anti-vaccine advocacy on the population in order to develop a program of further interventions to improve vaccination adherence.

The results of the opinion study of 358 people demonstrated that parents are extremely poorly aware of the problem of HPV infection, the associated risks, and the possibility of preventing diseases caused by HPV with vaccines. Only 21% of respondents know about the HPV problem and 31% have heard about vaccination. Only 49% of parents believe that it is necessary to vaccinate, but only 9% of respondents are ready to vaccinate their children. About 69% of parents doubt the need for vaccination, 22% categorically refused. Also, parents do not have exact knowledge at what age and who needs to be vaccinated, 63% believe that only girls need to be vaccinated, and 35% believe that adolescents of both sexes need to be vaccinated. For explanations about vaccination, 31% will turn to a pediatrician and 15% to a gynecologist; 39% prefer to study reviews on the Internet, and only 12% will receive information on official websites about vaccination.

The results of the opinion study of 254 doctors showed better awareness, and 83% gave a positive answer about the risks of HPV infection and the possibilities of vaccination; the most informed were obstetricians and gynecologists. The majority of doctors (98%) support vaccination, but only 50% are ready to vaccinate their child, 36% of them doubt the effectiveness, and 14% are not sure about the safety of vaccines, which also indicates a lack of knowledge. Obstetricians and gynecologists showed the highest adherence to HPV vaccination (86%). The majority of doctors are ready to receive additional information on vaccination of HPV-associated diseases from official sources: when contacting a polyclinic 59%; a skin and venereal dispensary, 21%; a pediatrician, 11%; an obstetrician-gynecologist, 28%, a dermatologist, 9%; and on official websites about vaccination—47%.

To raise awareness of the population and the medical community in our region, we have developed lectures and presentations for medical professionals and parents; created a video about vaccination, which was demonstrated in children's polyclinics; and developed and published booklets, posters, and leaflets for the population. Meetings were held with parents and teachers and medical workers in schools of the city, which were organized with the assistance of the Department of Education of KhMAO-Ugra. The text of the voluntary informed consent for parents has been developed, which includes all necessary information about the risk of HPV-associated diseases, the vaccination program and the effectiveness of immunization, and contraindications and possible postvaccination reactions. The introduction of such voluntary informed consent has increased the commitment of health professionals and parents to vaccination and reduced the frequency of refusals.

A "School of Health" is organized, where meetings with parents and schoolchildren are held on a regular basis. The objectives of this school are the following:

- Advocate to motivate vaccination and provide information on the risks of HPV infection and associated diseases

- Expose myths in order to gain the trust of parents and counter anti-vaccine agitation

- Persuade doubters on the example of highlighting the effectiveness of the regions where vaccination is carried out and familiarization with their own experience of vaccination in previous years in the KhMAO

- Live stream on Instagram account "School of Health"

Monitoring the effectiveness and safety of vaccines is an integral part of any vaccination program, which should be carried out both at the vaccination implementation stage and in the future.

Evaluation of the effectiveness of vaccination in the short term is traditionally carried out according to the incidence of genital warts, as the earliest marker of HPV infection.

HPV vaccination in the long term aims to reduce the incidence and mortality from cervical cancer, anal cancer, and other HPV-associated cancers. However, the introduction of a monitoring system, or register of vaccinated, will allow assessing not only the indicators of early effectiveness but also monitoring adverse events associated or not associated with vaccination.

Indicators such as a decrease in cases of genital warts or genital intraepithelial neoplasia in the vaccinated population will be recorded earlier than results in a decrease in HPV-associated cancers and may indicate the effectiveness of HPV vaccination.

For monitoring it is necessary to have a register of vaccinated. The creation of the register of vaccinated will allow assessing the following parameters: indicators of early effectiveness and monitoring adverse events associated and not associated with vaccination. The introduction of the HPV register should be carried out at all levels, from doctors involved in vaccination to health administrators involved in evaluating strategies to improve the health of citizens.

The information contained in the register will assess the following criteria for the implementation of the HPV vaccination program:

1. Accounting of vaccine coverage, age, and sex of the vaccinated. The ability to call adolescents for missed doses of the vaccine

2. Efficacy in reducing precancerous, cancerous, and other HPV-associated diseases: HPV infection; cervical and other HPV-associated genital neoplasia (CIN, AIN, VIN, VaIN); cervical cancer, adenocarcinoma in situ (AIS), anal cancer, vulvar cancer, and vaginal cancer; and anogenital warts

3. Monitoring adverse events related to vaccination time and distant in time

4. Modeling or correcting existing cervical cancer prevention screening programs

7. First results and expected effect of vaccination

The average age of development of cervical cancer and other HPV-associated cancers is 45 years, but it should be understood that cancer of the cervix, vulva, vagina, and anal canal is preceded by precancerous lesions, namely, cervical intraepithelial neoplasia 1/2/3 degree (CIN), adenocarcinoma in situ, vulvar and vaginal intraepithelial neoplasia (VIN, VaIN), and anal intraepithelial neoplasia (AIN), which occur at a younger age. The time required to develop cervical, vulvar, vaginal, and anal cancer from CIN, VIN, VaIN, AIN can take 9–15 years [1, 2].

International experts, including experts from the World Health Organization, agree that the ethical and time frame necessitates the use of precancerous lesions rather than cancer as the endpoint of HPV vaccination effectiveness. The ability of vaccination to effectively reduce precancerous lesions of the anogenital region in men and women suggests the absence of anogenital cancers in the future. Thus, the reduction of precancerous lesions of the anogenital region and the development of genital warts in women and men is recognized as the main marker for assessing the short- and medium-term effectiveness of HPV vaccination.

The economic damage of HPV in the Khanty-Mansiysk Autonomous Region-Ugra is about $5,730,000 per year.

Predicted effect of HPV-associated disease vaccination in KhMAO-Ugra:

- will be prevented by infection with human papillomavirus 6, 11, 16, and 18 types, which is not less than 99% of vaccinated teenagers due to development of postvaccinal immunity; this will prevent about 70% of all cervical cancer cases, 80% of cases of anal cancer, 60% of oropharyngeal cancer cases, 55% of cases of vaginal cancer, 48% of vulvar cancer cases, and 48% of cases of penile cancer.

- The incidence of genital warts will be reduced by at least 90% in the cohort (compared with unvaccinated groups) in the future 3–5 years.

- HPV vaccination will prevent costs by reducing the incidence of HPV in the amount of $3,900,000.

- Positive economic effect will be provided for the period of 5 years in the amount of $2,300,000, provided 70% vaccination coverage for girls 12 years in the Khanty-Mansiysk Autonomous Region-Ugra

- HPV vaccination will save 11,015 bed occupancy per year and prevent 101 deaths from malignant neoplasms per year.

When analyzing the incidence of HPV-associated diseases in KhMAO-Ugra, it was found that since 2011, the incidence of anogenital warts in adolescent girls has decreased both by the results of preventive examinations and by the incidence in the offices of a gynecologist. The incidence of HPV-associated diseases was monitored in a group of young women 8 and 10 years after vaccination. We examined 871 girls aged 20–22 who received vaccination at the age of 12 years old, and we did not register clinical manifestations of HPV infection (anogenital warts, CIN).

In addition, we noted the general population effect. The rate of primary incidence of anogenital warts in the adult population in KhMAO-Ugra for the period 2009–2008 decreased by 39%.

8. Conclusion

The lack of national HPV vaccination programs is not due to the lack of relevance of HPV-associated disease prevention but to the lack of sufficient financial resources to implement it. We hope that in the coming years, HPV vaccination will also be included in the Russian national vaccination calendar.

Factors that prevent the formation of recognition of vaccination are ignorance about HPV and cancer, lack of awareness of the risks of cancer, fears of undesirable consequences, and uncertainty about long-term vaccine protection. The effectiveness of HPV vaccination programs depends on the level of vaccination coverage, which in turn depends on the recognition of the importance of HPV vaccination by the government, health authorities, doctors, vaccinees, and their parents.

During vaccination, we should:

- Consider the possibility of protection against the largest range of HPV-associated cancer and other diseases, that is, use at least quadrivalent HPV vaccine with inclusion in the vaccination program for boys aged 12–14.

- Achieve vaccination coverage for at least 70% of girls aged 12–13.

- Implement a system to monitor the effectiveness of the vaccination program, including short-, medium-, and long-term indicators.

It is necessary to work on the improvement of professional training of health workers in preventing communicable diseases—organization of thematic conferences and round tables and development of thematic improvement of doctors and nurses.

We see the need to continue to work to provide the public with reliable and objective information on vaccination.

In order to promote vaccination and improve its effectiveness, further activities should be undertaken with the involvement of the pediatric care service under the immunization program:

- Conduct field meetings with parents, representatives of schools, and children's clinics.

- Continue explanatory work in mass media in connection with high activity of anti-vaccine agitation on the Internet.

- Prepare booklets with questions on reproductive health, develop volunteer movement among students, and conduct surveys of young people.

Author details

Larisa Dmitrievna Belotserkovtseva* and Yulia Igorevna Mayer
Surgut Clinical Perinatal Center, Surgut State University, KhMAO-Ugra, Russia

*Address all correspondence to: mayerjul@gmail.com

References

[1] The WHO Position Paper on Vaccines against Human Papillomavirus (HPV). 2009. Available from: http://www.who.int/immunization/documents/HPV_position_paper_summary.pdf?ua=1

[2] Human Papillomavirus and Related Diseases Report/World/Version. 2014. Available from: www.hpvcenter.net

[3] Munoz N, et al. HPV in the Etiology of Human Cancer. Vaccine 24S3. 2006. S3/1–S3/10

[4] Kyrgiou M, Koliopoulos G, Martin-Hirsch P, et al. Obstetric outcomes after conservative treatment for intraepithelial or early invasive cervical lesions: Systematic review and meta-analysis. Lancet. 2006;**367**:489-498

[5] GLOBOCAN. WHO/ICO Information Centre on HPV and Cervical Cancer (HPV Information Centre). Human Papillomavirus and Related Cancers in World. Summary. Available from: www.who.int/hpvcentre [Accessed: September 09, 2012]

[6] Kostin AA. Analysis of statistical data on malignant neoplasms associated with human papilloma virus. Research and Practical Medicine Journal. 2016;**3**:66-78

[7] Gretsova OP, Kostin AA, et al. Morbidity and mortality from malignant neoplasms associated with human papilloma virus. Research and Practical Medicine Journal. 2017;**4**(3):33-50

[8] Kaprin AD, et al. The State of Cancer Care in Russia in 2018. Moscow. 2019. Available from: http://www.oncology.ru/service/statistics/condition/2018.pdf

[9] Tikhomirov AL et al. Human papilloma virus: From understanding of immunopathogenesis to rational tactics of management. Gynecology. 2018;**20**(3):5-11

[10] The State of Cancer Care to the Population of Khanty-Mansiysk Autonomous Region -Ugra in 2018. Khanty-Mansiysk: Medical Information and Analytical Center. 2018. Available from: https://www.dzhmao.ru/company/zdorove-v-tsifrakh/pokazateli-zabolevaemosti.php

[11] Evstigneeva NP. Expression of oncoprotein E7 in patients with urogenital papillomavirus infection. Russian Journal of Skin and Venereal Diseases. 2006;**2**:4-6

[12] Kondrikov NI. Others the importance of immunohistochemical determination of biomarkers of squamous epithelial lesions of the cervix. Obstetrics and Gynecology. 2010;**6**:44-48

[13] Belotserkovtseva LD et al. Reproductive behavior of adolescents and experience in prevention of HPV-associated diseases in KHMAO-Ugra. Questions of Gynecology, Obstetrics and Perinatology. 2018;**17**(1):100-108

[14] Kumykova ZH. Human papillomavirus vaccines: Analysis of efficacy and safety of use. Reproductive Health of Children and Adolescents. 2015;**3**:9-18

[15] The Integrated Fight against Cervical Cancer. Clinical Guideline. 2nd ed. Geneva: World health organisation; 2014. p. 364

[16] Federal Clinical Guidelines for the Management of Patients with Anogenital (Venereal) Warts. Moscow; 2015. p. 14

[17] Vaccination of diseases caused by human papilloma virus: Federal Clinical Recommendations of the Ministry of Health of the Russian Federation,

The Union of Pediatricians of Russia. Moscow: Pediatrician; 2016. p. 40

[18] Introduction of HPV Vaccines in EU Countries—An Update. Stockholm: ECDC. 2012. Available from: http://www.ecdc.europa.eu/en/publications/publications/20120905_gui_hpv_vaccine_update.pdf

[19] Bosch FX et al. Reframing cervical cancer prevention. Expanding the field towards prevention of human papillomavirus infections and related diseases. Vaccine. 2012;**30**(Suppl 5):F1-F11

[20] Stanley M. Nature. 2012;**488**:S10

[21] European Centre for Disease Control and Prevention (ECDC). The Introduction of HPV Vaccines in the EU is an Update. Stockholm: ECDC. 2012. Available from: http://www.ecdc.europa.eu/en/publications/publications/20120905_gui_hpv_vaccine_update.pdf

[22] Baranov AA et al. Analysis of economic and social demographic burden of HPV-associated diseases and economic efficiency of HPV vaccination in Russia. Pediatric Pharmacology. 2019;**16**(2):101-110

[23] Grulich AE, et al. Quadrivalent HPV Vaccination and Genital Warts in Australia, 2004-2010. O-04.01. Abstract book IPV 2011

[24] Baandrup L et al. Significant decrease in the incidence of genital warts in young Danish women after implementation of a national human papillomavirus vaccination program. Sexually Transmitted Diseases. 2013;**40**:130-135

[25] Hammad A et al. Decline in in-patient treatments of genital warts among young Australians following the national HPV vaccination program. BMC Infectious Diseases. 2013;**13**:140

[26] Bresse X, Goergen C, Prager B, Joura E. Universal vaccination with the quadrivalent HPV vaccine in Austria: Impact on virus circulation, public health and cost-effectiveness analysis. Expert Review of Pharmacoeconomics & Outcomes Research. 2014;**14**:269-281

[27] Bresse X, Cassel T, Adam M. Universal Vaccination against 6/11/16/18 HPV-related diseases in Sweden: towards HPV disease control? EUROGIN 2013 European Research Organization on Genital Infection and Neoplasia 2013 International Multidisciplinary Congress. Florence, Italy. Abstract P 3-3

[28] Kothari S, Nwankwo C, Pillsbury M. The health and economic impact of a quadrivalent human papillomavirus vaccine (6/11/16/18) in Columbia: A transmission dynamic model-based evaluation. Value in Health. 2013;**16**(7):A713

[29] Инструкция по применению вакцины Гардасил. 2013г. Сайт ГРЛС. http://grls.rosminzdrav.ru/InstrImgMZ.aspx?isNew=1&idReg=36102&page=6&isOld=1&t=c650f4d1-cf75-4957-93d0-dc72436e30cd

[30] Zarochentseva NV et al. Preventive vaccination against cervical cancer and HPV-associated disorders: International and national data/gynecology. Endocrinology. 2018;**146**(2):52-58

[31] Arbyn M et al. Prophylactic vaccination against human papillomaviruses to prevent cervical cancer and its precursors. Cochrane Database of Systematic Reviews. 2018;**5**:CD009069. DOI: 10.1002/14651858.CD009069.pub3

[32] FUTURE I/II Study Group. Four year efficacy of prophylactic human papillomavirus quadrivalent vaccine against low grade cervical, vulvar, and vaginal intraepithelial neoplasia

and anogenital warts: Randomised controlled trial. BMJ. 2010;**340**:c3493

[33] Donovan B et al. Quadrivalent human papillomavirus vaccination and trends in genital warts in Australia: Analysis of national sentinel surveillance data. The Lancet Infectious Diseases. 2011;**11**:39-44

Chapter 2

HPV-Positive Oral Squamous Cell Carcinoma

Șerban Vifor Gabriel Bertești eanu, Raluca Grigore, Alexandru Nicolaescu and Mihnea Cojocărița-Condeescu

Abstract

Head and neck malignancies represent the sixth most frequent type of cancer currently in worldwide statistics. Of these, oral and pharyngeal cancers have steadily increased, being linked with the increase in HPV infection pandemic. This rise is not due to one cause, but rather multiple factors such as lifestyle and sexual behavior pattern changes and globalization. Because of the anatomy of the oral cavity and oropharynx, the proper diagnosis is easily delayed, and patients present with advanced stage disease, which requires aggressive and extensive surgery along with neck dissection and chemoradiotherapy. Patients with advanced stage disease have a high recurrence risk with a low 5-year survival rate. Preventing the HPV infection is of course desirable, but right now, for adults which already are infected and have a higher risk of developing HPV-related neoplasias, as well as for our head and neck cancer patients, alternative treatment algorithms are necessary.

Keywords: head and neck cancer, HPV, OPSCC, oral cancer, neck dissection

1. Introduction

Head and neck squamous cell carcinoma (HNSCC) is the sixth most common malignancy in the world [1]. The tonsils are the most common location in oropharyngeal malignancy. Despite being easily accessible to examination, its symptoms are usually ignored especially in early stages, leading to high morbidity and mortality. Traditionally oral and oropharyngeal cancers were attributed to smoking and alcohol abuse, but in more recent years there has been an increase in numbers due to high prevalence of Human papillomavirus (HPV) infection. The presence of HPV can alter the prognosis of the disease, and recently there was a change in the WHO classifications and TNM staging to reflect this [2]. Depending on the stage of the disease, treatment for oral and oropharyngeal cancers consists of surgery and/or chemoradiotherapy.

2. Etiology

Traditionally smoking is considered the major factor in developing tonsil cancer. More than three quarters of oropharyngeal cancers are associated with tobacco use in all its forms (cigarettes, cigars, pipes, chewed tobacco). Secondhand smokers also have an increased risk of developing head and neck cancers. Alcohol is the second major risk factor in the etiology of tonsil cancer. Although studies have not shown a direct link between the use of alcohol alone in carcinogenesis, the combined effect of tobacco and alcohol has a synergic effect on the development of cancer cells [3].

In the last 10 years, HPV infection has been widely recognized as an important etiological factor in the development of head and neck squamous cell carcinomas. The development of PCR analysis or in situ hybridization has demonstrated the impact of HPV in oropharyngeal malignancy [1]. Gillison [4] was the first to show that HPV-positive oropharyngeal cancers have different molecular, clinical, and pathological traits than HPV-negative cancers. Although HPV is considered to play a vital role in most head and neck cancers, studies have only proven its impact in oropharyngeal cancers [5].

HPV is a double-stranded DNA oncovirus and is epitheliotropic, infecting the basal cells of the epithelium and can be found in up to 60% of squamous cell carcinomas of the oropharynx [6]. There are more than 150 isolated strains of HPV, but only two types 16 and 18 are most commonly linked to oropharyngeal cancers. The oncogenic effect of HPV is due to two proteins E6 and E7 that target the p53 and pRB (retinoblastoma) tumor suppressor genes of the infected cells making them vulnerable to mutations [7]. The loss of the pRB tumor suppressor determines the intranuclear accumulation of p16. p16 has a tumor suppressor role which normally would inhibit cell cycle but is overexpressed in HPV-positive tumors due to the action of E7. It is considered a useful marker in oropharyngeal cancers [8]. Due to the large body of evidence that suggest that HPV-positive and HPV-negative oropharyngeal cancers represent distinct subgroups of OPSCC, the National Comprehensive Cancer Network (NCCN) guidelines as of 2017 require HPV testing for all oropharyngeal tumors and that the HPV status must be included as a stratification factor [2]. The latest staging for oropharyngeal cancers takes into account the distinct groups of OPSCC, and because HPV-positive cancers tend to have a better prognosis, separate TNM staging systems are used [9, 10].

Dietary habits also play a role in carcinogenesis although harder to properly quantify. For example, iron deficiency may lead to an increased vulnerability of the oropharyngeal mucosa and decreased immune system. A diet low in fruits and vegetables can lead to a vitamin A and vitamin E deficiency that is associated with an increased risk of developing oropharyngeal malignancies. Poor oral hygiene can also be a risk factor especially for tobacco and alcohol users [11].

3. Symptoms and diagnosis

Oropharyngeal cancer is usually located in the tonsillar fossa, but extension to adjacent structures is common (**Figure 1**). Frequently tonsillar carcinoma extends downward to the tongue base along the glosso-tonsillar sulcus (**Figure 2**) and to the soft palate laterally. Laterally the tonsillar fossa is bounded by the superior constrictor muscle of the pharynx which offers some resistance to the spread of carcinoma. Extension past the superior constrictor muscle represents involvement of the parapharyngeal space with consecutive involvement of the pterygoid musculature or mandible locally advanced disease. Extension to the skull base is rare but possible.

Due to its rich lymphatic drainage, lymph node involvement is present in about 70% of patients. The most common lymph node levels affected are level II and level III [12].

Distant metastasis from tonsillar cancer occurs in about 15–30% of cases; the most common sites are the lung, liver, and bones [13].

Tonsillar cancer may present with a variety of signs and symptoms. In the early stages, the patient is usually asymptomatic, or it can mimic some mild diseases like sore throat or acute tonsillitis. Patients usually complain of sore throat, unilateral

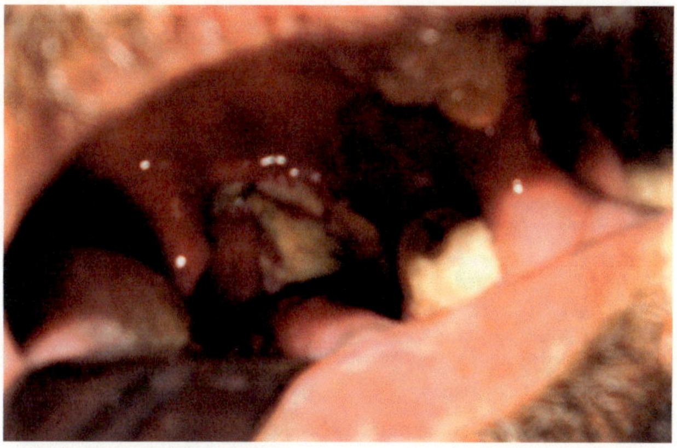

Figure 1.
Oral examination of a male patient with a left oropharyngeal tumor which infiltrates and deforms the tonsillar fossa as well as part of the soft palate, with ulceration and suprainfection.

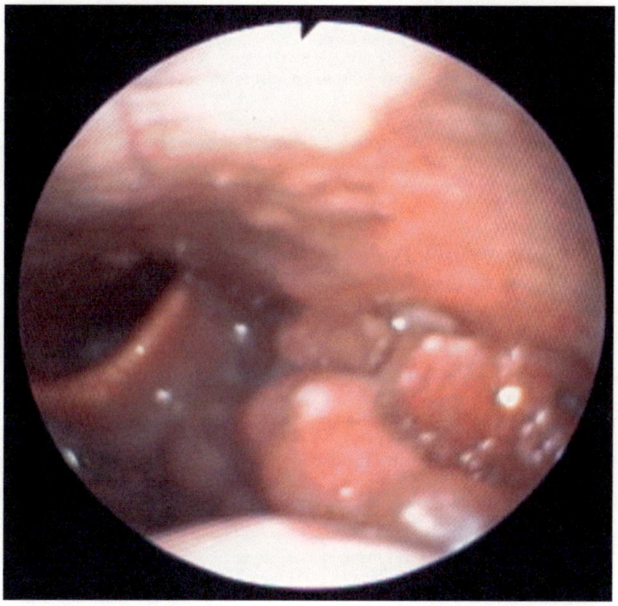

Figure 2.
Fiber-optic endoscopy of a male patient showing inferior spread of a left side oropharyngeal tumor towards the tongue base.

otalgia, or a feeling of a mass in the throat. In advanced stages it can present with dysphagia. In latter stages the patient may present with trismus or bleeding from the mouth. If the tumor has ulcerations and necrosis, patients will usually complain of bad breath. The rich lymphatic drainage could mean that the first sign of disease is enlarged lymph nodes especially in the jugulodigastric region (group II). Such patients must be asked about weight loss, hoarseness, and odynophagia. A thorough patient history about tobacco and alcohol use and other known etiological factors (including known HPV infection) may raise suspicion of a malignant tumor. HPV-positive tumors will typically appear in younger nonsmoking patients.

Patients diagnosed with a tumor involving the oral and oropharyngeal regions must undergo a full ENT examination, with neck palpation, flexible endoscopy, and biopsy. After histological confirmation of the malignancy, imaging studies must be obtained to stage the tumor. Contrast CT scans represent the standard method for

Stage	T	N	M
I	T0-T2	N0	M0
	T0-T2	N1	M0
II	T0-T2	N2	M0
	T3	N0-N2	M0
III	T0-T3	N3	M0
	T4	N0-N3	
IV	T Any	N Any	M1

Table 1.
AJCC staging of HPV-positive (p16+) oropharyngeal cancer [14].

Tumor	Characteristics
T0	No primary tumor identified
T1	Tumor less than 2 cm in any dimension
T2	Tumor between 2 and 4 cm
T3	Tumor greater than 4 cm in any dimension or extension to lingual surface of the epiglottis
T4	= moderately advanced local disease—tumor invades the larynx, extrinsic muscles of the tongue, medial pterygoid muscles, hard palate, mandible or beyond

Table 2.
AJCC tumor characteristics regarding HPV-positive (p16+) oropharyngeal carcinoma [14].

Lymph node (N)	Clinical N (cN)	Pathological N (pN)
Nx	Regional lymph nodes cannot be assessed	Regional lymph nodes cannot be assessed
N0	No regional lymph node metastasis	No regional lymph node metastasis
N1	One or more ipsilateral lymph nodes, none >6 cm	Metastasis in 4 or fewer lymph nodes
N2	Contralateral or bilateral lymph nodes, none >6 cm	Metastasis in more than 4 lymph nodes
N3	Lymph node(s) > 6 cm	

Table 3.
AJCC lymph node characteristics for staging of disease regarding HPV-positive (p16+) oropharyngeal cancer.

staging and should include the skull base, cervical region, thorax, and abdomen to possibly identify secondary tumors. Contrast-enhanced MRI is superior to CT in detecting soft tissue extension and involvement but may be influenced by dental foreign materials.

Staging of the disease is done by using the AJCC cancer staging system (**Table 1**) that uses three variables—primary tumor characteristics (T), lymph node involvement (N), and the existence of metastases (M).

Starting from 1 January 2017, all patients with oropharyngeal cancer should be tested for the presence of HPV, thus classifying them in one of two possible categories—HPV positive ($p16^{INK4A}$+) and HPV negative. There is no current gold standard test, because all available testing methods were developed for cervical cancer, and not perfectly adapted for tonsillar cancer. However, p16 protein IHC is currently used for detecting HPV presence [15].

Tumor and lymph node characteristics are described in **Tables 2** and **3**, whereas the presence of distant metastases automatically stages the disease into the last and most severe stage—stage IV (**Table 1**).

4. Treatment and outcome

Treatment of oropharyngeal malignancy depends on the disease stage, but the principle that guides it is the same as in all cancer surgery: local disease control. Thus, with modern surgical and irradiation techniques, 5-year survival rates of almost 100% are attainable [16].

For the purpose of management protocol, oropharyngeal cancer is divided into early-stage (T1 and T2) and advanced diseases (T3 and T4). The latter are divided into resectable and non-resectable tumors. According to this, treatment for early-stage disease should be either surgery or radiation therapy with concurrent chemotherapy. Surgical treatment consists of excision of the primary tumor, either by a trans-oral approach or by external approach (lateral pharyngotomy or trans-mandibular approach by mandibular swing technique (**Figures 3–5**)).

Most oropharyngeal tumors are accessible by trans-oral approach. This is the least aggressive type of surgical approach, with the least morbidity. Auto-static mouth gags (McIver, Dingmann, etc.) permit good exposure of the surgical site, and excision by electrocautery, radiofrequency, and CO_2 laser, and optical augmentation either using surgical loupes or operating microscopes permit tackling most of the T1 to T3 tumors [17].

Tumors extending downward to the epiglottis and hypopharynx (pyriform sinus) require an external approach, by lateral pharyngotomy. This approach provides access to the oro- and hypopharynx, as well as control of the cervical large blood vessels and lymph nodes [18–20].

Advanced tumors (T4), tumors which involve adjacent structures (extrinsic muscles of the tongue, larynx, mandible, pterygoid muscles, or hard palate), often require an even more aggressive external approach—by lateral mandibulotomy—the so-called mandibular swing technique. This approach permits access to the

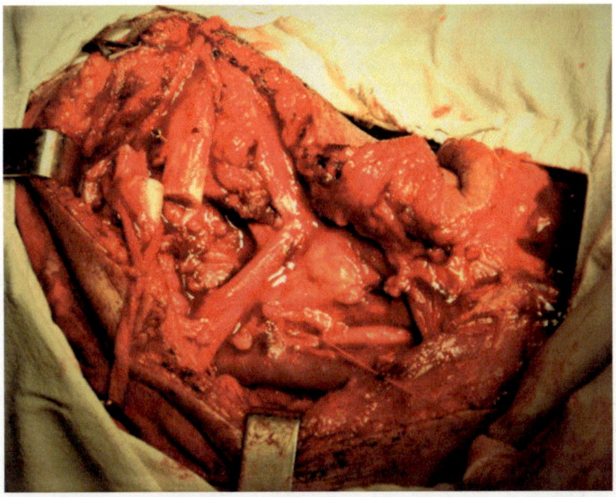

Figure 3.
External approach to a right side advanced (T4) oropharyngeal cancer which shows the neck dissection, with internal jugular vein and bifurcation of the common carotid artery visible inferior to the posterior belly of the omohyoid muscle, as well as the mandibulotomy—The creation of the mandibular "swing."

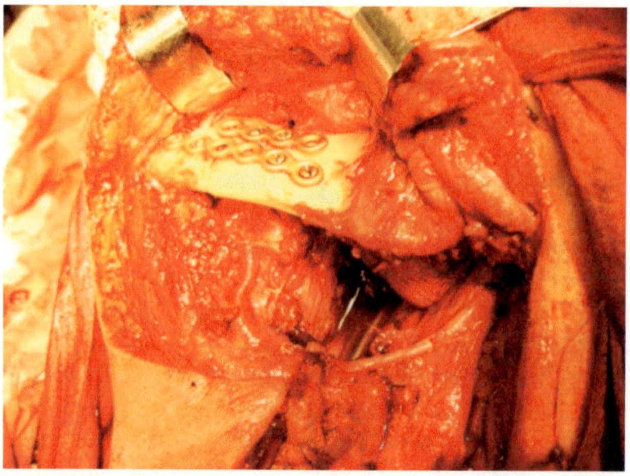

Figure 4.
External approach to a left side advanced oropharyngeal tumor, via mandibular "swing" demonstrating closure of the mandibulotomy using two titanium miniplates anchored with screws.

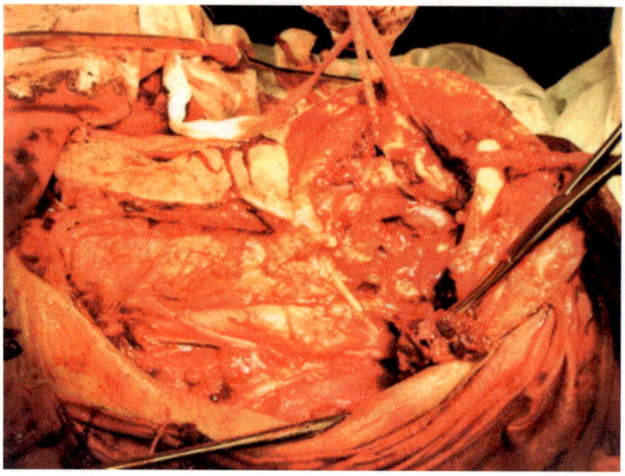

Figure 5.
Extensive external approach to a left side advanced (T4) tumor of the oropharynx and hypopharynx extending to the bony cortex of the mandible—with modified radical neck dissection and lateral mandibulotomy, with the two resulting mandibular pieces being pulled apart at different angles so as to permit wider access.

oral cavity, oropharynx, as well as hypopharynx and lateral cervical lymph nodes, parapharyngeal space, and masticator space and allows instrumentation of the entire oral cavity, making hard palate resections possible [21, 22].

Whichever surgical approach to the primary tumor the surgeon opts for, just as important as the complete excision of the tumor (the T) is the neck dissection. Tumors that do not pass the midline usually require ipsilateral lymph node dissection. However, bilateral neck dissection is sometimes required because of the vast network of lymphatics that drain the lateral pharyngeal area—most patients present with at least clinically N1 on diagnosis [23, 24].

The alternative to surgical excision of the tumor is external intensity-modulated radiation therapy (IMRT) with or without adjuvant chemotherapy. This procedure has similar outcomes compared to surgery in cases of early-stage tumors but is slightly inferior compared to surgery when addressing advanced tumors. The dose delivered to the surrounding tissues is responsible for the toxicity and late adverse effects of radiation therapy, such as osteoradionecrosis of the mandible, radiomucositis, xerostomia, dental cavities, and teeth avulsion [25]. These have a high impact on the patients' quality of life; thus modern management of HPV-positive oropharyngeal cancer consists in trans-oral excision (with a rising trend towards robotic surgery) of the primary tumor with selective neck dissection followed by low-dose radiation therapy [25].

5. Conclusions

As HPV infection is a growing concern worldwide, cases of HPV-positive oral and oropharyngeal carcinoma become more frequently encountered. Treatment options for this type of malignancy follow the same principles as for non-HPV-positive squamous cell carcinoma of the oral cavity and pharynx, consisting in surgery for locoregional control of the primary tumor and regional lymph nodes and radiation therapy—either as a stand-alone option or as an adjuvant therapy following surgical excision.

However, particularities of HPV-positive oropharyngeal cancer have led to a separation of this pathologic entity from the rest of squamous cell carcinomas involving the oropharynx. These tumors have a better outcome following treatment and thus treatment options were de-escalated to offer the same outcome and 5-year survival as well as less morbidity and a better quality of life.

New perspectives in treating the chronic HPV infection as well as preventing this infection by introducing efficient vaccination programs that target girls and boys also offer a positive future perspective on reducing malignancies associated with this viral infection, including those affecting the oral cavity and pharynx.

Author details

Șerban Vifor Gabriel Berteșteanu[1,2], Raluca Grigore[1,2], Alexandru Nicolaescu[1*] and Mihnea Cojocărița-Condeescu[1]

1 ENT Head and Neck Surgery Department, General Medicine Faculty, "Carol Davila" University of Medicine and Pharmacy, Bucharest, Romania

2 ENT Head and Neck Surgery Clinic, "Colțea" Clinical Hospital Bucharest, Bucharest, Romania

*Address all correspondence to: alexandru87nicolaescu@gmail.com

References

[1] Chaturvedi AK, Engels EA, Pfeiffer RM, Hernandez BY, Xiao W, Kim E, et al. Human papillomavirus and rising oropharyngeal cancer incidence in the United States. Journal of Clinical Oncology. 2011;**29**(32):4294-4301

[2] Adelstein D, Gillison ML, Pfister DG, Spencer S, Adkins D, Brizel DM, et al. NCCN guidelines insights: Head and neck cancers, version 2.2017. Journal of the National Comprehensive Cancer Network. 2017;**15**(6):761-770

[3] Morse DE, Psoter WJ, Cleveland D, Cohen D, Mohit-Tabatabai M, Kosis DL, et al. Smoking and drinking in relation to oral cancer and oral epithelial dysplasia. Cancer Causes & Control. 2007;**18**(9):919-929

[4] Gillison ML. Human papillomavirus-associated head and neck cancer is a distinct epidemiologic, clinical, and molecular entity. Seminars in Oncology. 2004;**31**(6):744-754

[5] Stransky N, Egloff AM, Tward AD, Kostic AD, Cibulskis K, Sivachenko A, et al. The mutational landscape of head and neck squamous cell carcinoma. Science. 2011;**333**(6046):1157-1160

[6] Kreimer AR, Clifford GM, Boyle P, Franceschi S. Human papillomavirus types in head and neck squamous cell carcinomas worldwide: A systematic review. Cancer Epidemiology, Biomarkers & Prevention. 2005;**14**(2):467-475. Available from: http://www.ncbi.nlm.nih.gov/pubmed/15734974 [Accessed: 3 May 2019]

[7] Hassani S, Castillo A, Ohori JI, Higashi M, Kurono Y, Akiba S, et al. Molecular pathogenesis of human papillomavirus type 16 in tonsillar squamous cell carcinoma. Anticancer Research. 2015;**35**(12):6633-6638. Available from: www.iiar-anticancer.org [Accessed: 10 December 2019]

[8] Oh JE, Kim JO, Shin JY, Zhang XH, Won HS, Chun SH, et al. Molecular genetic characterization of p53 mutated oropharyngeal squamous cell carcinoma cells transformed with human papillomavirus E6 and E7 oncogenes. International Journal of Oncology. 2013;**43**(2):383-393

[9] Oral Cavity and Oropharyngeal Cancer Stages [Internet]. Available from: https://www.cancer.org/cancer/oral-cavity-and-oropharyngeal-cancer/detection-diagnosis-staging/staging.html [Accessed: 10 December 2019]

[10] Pfister DG, Spencer S, Adelstein D, Adkins D, Brizel D. NCCN Clinical Practice Guidelines in Oncology: Head and Neck Cancers [Internet]. 2.2017. 2017. Available from: https://www.nccn.org/professionals/physician_gls/pdf/head-and-neck.pdf

[11] Gupta B, Bray F, Kumar N, Johnson NW. Associations between oral hygiene habits, diet, tobacco and alcohol and risk of oral cancer: A case-control study from India. Cancer Epidemiology. 2017;**51**:7-14

[12] Lee DJ, Kwon MJ, Nam ES, Kwon JH, Kim JH, Rho YS, et al. Histopathologic predictors of lymph node metastasis and prognosis in tonsillar squamous cell carcinoma. Korean Journal of Pathology. 2013;**47**(3):203-210. Available from: https://www.ncbi.nlm.nih.gov/pmc/articles/PMC3701815/ [Accessed: 17 December 2019]

[13] Chung TS, Stefani S. Distant metastases of carcinoma of tonsillar region: A study of 475 patients. Journal of Surgical Oncology. 1980;**14**(1):5-9. Available from: http://www.ncbi.nlm.nih.gov/pubmed/7382512 [Accessed: 17 December 2019]

[14] Lydiatt W, O'Sullivan B, Patel S. Major changes in head and neck staging

for 2018. American Society of Clinical Oncology Educational Book. 2018;**38**(38):505-514. Available from: http://ascopubs.org/doi/10.1200/EDBK_199697 [Accessed: 17 December 2019]

[15] Kim KY, Lewis JS, Chen Z. Current status of clinical testing for human papillomavirus in oropharyngeal squamous cell carcinoma. The Journal of Pathology: Clinical Research. 2018;**4**:213-226. Available from: http://www.ncbi.nlm.nih.gov/pubmed/30058293 [Accessed: 17 December 2019]

[16] Foote RL, Hilgenfeld RU, Kunselman SJ, Schaid DJ, Buskirk SJ, Grado GL, et al. Radiation therapy for squamous cell carcinoma of the tonsil. Mayo Clinic Proceedings. 1994;**69**(6):525-531. Available from: http://www.ncbi.nlm.nih.gov/pubmed/8189757 [Accessed: 19 December 2019]

[17] Flint PW, Haughey BH, Lund VJ, Niparko JK, Robbins TK, Thomas RJ, et al. Cummings Otolaryngology—Head and Neck Surgery. 6th ed. Philadelphia, PA: Saunders-Elsevier; 2015. DOI: 10.1016/B978-0-323-05283-2.00009-4

[18] Bertolin A, Ghirardo G, Lionello M, Giacomelli L, Lucioni M, Rizzotto G. Lateral pharyngotomy approach in the treatment of oropharyngeal carcinoma. European Archives of Oto-Rhino-Laryngology. 2017;**274**(6):2573-2580

[19] Laccourreye O, Benito J, Menard M, Garcia D, Malinvaud D, Holsinger C. Lateral pharyngotomy for selected invasive squamous cell carcinoma of the lateral oropharynx—Part I: How. Laryngoscope. 2013;**123**(11):2712-2717

[20] Laccourreye O, Seccia V, Ménard M, Garcia D, Vacher C, Holsinger FC. Extended lateral pharyngotomy for selected squamous cell carcinomas of the lateral tongue base. The Annals of Otology, Rhinology, and Laryngology. 2009;**118**(6):428-434

[21] Spiro RH, Gerold FP, Strong EW. Mandibular "swing" approach for oral and oropharyngeal tumors. Head & Neck Surgery. 1981;**3**(5):371-378. Available from: http://doi.wiley.com/10.1002/hed.2890030505 [Accessed: 19 December 2019]

[22] Holsinger FC, Laccourreye O, Weber RS. Surgical approaches for cancer of the oropharynx. Operative Techniques in Otolaryngology-Head and Neck Surgery. 2005;**16**(1 Spec. Iss):40-48. Available from: https://www.sciencedirect.com/science/article/abs/pii/S1043181005000023 [Accessed: 19 December 2019]

[23] Goudakos JK, Markou K, Nikolaou A, Themelis C, Vital V. Management of the clinically negative neck (N0) of supraglottic laryngeal carcinoma: A systematic review. European Journal of Surgical Oncology. 2009;**35**:223-229

[24] Zenga J, Stadler M, Massey B, Campbell B, Shukla M, Awan M, et al. Lymph node yield from neck dissection in HPV-associated oropharyngeal cancer. Laryngoscope. 2019. Available from: http://www.ncbi.nlm.nih.gov/pubmed/31206708 [Accessed: 19 December 2019]

[25] De Felice F, Tombolini V, Valentini V, De Vincentiis M, Mezi S, Brugnoletti O, et al. Advances in the management of HPV-related oropharyngeal cancer. Journal of Oncology. 2019;**2019**:9173729. Available from: http://www.ncbi.nlm.nih.gov/pubmed/31097964 [Accessed: 19 December 2019]

Chapter 3

Human Papillomavirus Infection: Management and Treatment

Suchibrata Das

Abstract

Human papillomavirus infections are very common and recurrent. Their presentation varies according to their site of affection. Spontaneous recovery is common in a good number of patients. An ideal wart therapy resolves all or maximum number of warts, is painless, needs only one or a part of a wart treated, needs only minimum number of treatments, leaves no scar, offers lifetime HPV immunity and is easily available for all patients. Various modalities of treatment are available—from some folk and alternative therapies to destructive, antimitotic, virucidal, immunotherapy and combination of therapies. In every modality, the result is significant. Younger individuals with short duration of illness usually have the highest clearance rates for various treatments. Recurrence rate is also high in almost every treatment modality. Immunotherapy has a promising role.

Keywords: human papillomavirus infection, chemical cautery, electrocautery, cryotherapy, laser therapy, immunotherapy

1. Introduction

Human papillomaviruses (HPVs) are a large and diverse group of viruses with 174 completely characterised types, with new HPV types being continuously found [1]. There are five major HPV genera: *Alphapapillomavirus*, *Betapapillomavirus*, Gamma papillomavirus, Mu papillomavirus and Nu papillomavirus. HPVs infect epithelial cells in genital mucosa (*Alphapapillomaviruses* only), oral mucosa or skin (representatives of all five genera). The most common clinical manifestation is verruca, with different morphological forms. The histology shows acanthosis, elongation of dermal papillae, presence of vacuolated cells and koilocytes. Subclinical manifestations are invisible to the human eye. These subclinical lesions are flat and multiple. Their clinical insignificance facilitates their spread, and in women their persistence is possibly related to genital cancer.

2. Diagnosis

2.1 Clinical diagnosis

The clinical picture of cutaneous warts differs by specific location on the body [2]. Most extragenital warts are benign, and usually clinical diagnosis is adequate, but sometimes additional methods are required especially in atypical, subclinical or dysplastic lesions. Genital lesions are more prone to transform to malignancy, so determining the extent of disease is essential. Examining the wart and scraping off the top layer of the wart to check for signs of dark, pinpoint dots—clotted blood vessels—are common with warts.

2.2 Dermatoscopy

Warts can be visualised exceptionally well by dermoscopy, especially the black dots. Dermoscopy is also very useful in terms of differential diagnosis and follow-up [2].

2.3 Acetowhitening

Genital/mucosal lesions remain undetected for a long time; not only that, all lesions may not be clinically evident at a time. Topical application of 3–5% of acetic acid for 3–5 min and followed by examination with 10X hand lens or colposcope is a reasonable accurate diagnostic tool. Lesions will be represented as tiny white papules. The routine use of this procedure to detect mucosal changes attributed to HPV infection is not recommended because the results do not influence clinical management.

3. Laboratory investigations

3.1 Histology

Acanthosis, epidermal hyperplasia, papillomatosis, compact orthokeratosis, hypergranulosis, tortuous dermal papillary capillaries, and vertical tiers of parakeratotic cells are the typical histological findings of warts. In the granular layer, cells have coarse keratohyalin granules and vacuoles surrounding wrinkled-appearing nuclei. Koilocytes are pathognomonic.

3.2 Immunohistochemistry or immunocytochemistry using type-common and type-specific antibodies

3.2.1 DNA in situ hybridization

In situ hybridization is a direct signal detection assay. It preserves the morphological context with HPV DNA signals. It has low sensitivity; however, in recent years, using improved signal-detecting method, sensitivity increased. It is becoming a valuable screening tool for women of age more than 30 years.

3.3 Polymer-based enzyme-linked immunosorbent assay (ELISA) for immunoglobulin G (IgG) antibody (Ab) against HPV 16 capsid

3.3.1 PCR for HPV DNA

Patients who are diagnosed with condylomata need a Papanicolaou (Pap) test of the cervix in accordance with the guidelines of the American College of Obstetricians and Gynaecologists

Computed tomography (CT) or magnetic resonance imaging (MRI) can be used to determine the extent of spread of cervical carcinoma and extensive anogenital papillomatosis that has spread into the pelvis.

4. Treatment

Warts are usually self-limiting. Large studies have shown complete spontaneous remission in 42% of patients after 2 months; in 53%, after 6 months; and in 65%, after 2 years [2]. The intact immune system plays the most important role for preventing HPV infection. This can be seen in patients with primary immunodeficiency or in immunosuppressed patients.

HPV-induced warts are the most common skin disorder in organ transplant recipients [3]. Children with recalcitrant extragenital wart may suffer from primary immunodeficiency. It has been shown that immunosuppressed patients experience resolution of treatment-refractory warts once their immune status has improved [4]. The known spontaneous remission of HPV-induced warts, which is attributed to cell-bound mechanisms, underscores the role of the immune system, including an increase in Th1 cytokines and infiltration of T cells ($CD4^+$, $CD8^+$) around the diseased tissue [5].

Guidelines for the management of cutaneous warts have been prepared for dermatologists on behalf of the British Association of Dermatologists [6]. The guideline highlighted the ideal aims of treatment of warts as follows: (i) Removal of wart without recurrence. (ii) Treatment should result with no scars. (iii) Immunity that induced by treatment should be lifelong [5]. The general principles observed in the treatment of warts are the following: (1) There is no need to treat all warts. (2) Treatment indications are pain, interference with function, cosmetic embarrassment and risk of malignancy. (3) All the treatments have success rate not very high (average 60 ± 70% clearance in 3 months). (4) An immune response is usually essential for clearance. Immunocompromised individuals may never show wart clearance. (5) Younger individuals with short duration of illness usually have the highest clearance rates for various treatments [5].

There is a high rate of spontaneous remission, especially in children, so 'wait-and-see' approach is feasible in many cases. Regular filing or paring down the hyperkeratotic layer makes the lesion thin and comfortable. Simple measure to limit the spread of lesion should be encouraged. The treatment of warts can be broadly classified into destructive, antimitotic, virucidal, immunotherapy, and some folk and alternative therapies which have recently become popular again.

The goals of wart treatment are to resolve all or a maximum number of warts, make it painless, need only one or a part of a wart treated, only need minimum number of treatments, leave no scar, offer lifetime HPV immunity and be easily available for all patients [7]. The criteria for wart treatment, developed by the American Academy of Dermatology in 1995, [7] include (1) the patient's desire for therapy; (2) symptoms of pain, bleeding, itching or burning; (3) disabling or disfiguring lesions; (4) large numbers or large sizes of lesions; (5) the patient's desire to prevent the spread of warts to unblemished skin of self or others; and (6) an immunocompromised condition [6].

4.1 Destructive therapy

The lesions are damaged or removed by different procedures followed by clinical cure. The destructive therapies include surgical removal by curettage and cautery, chemical cautery, cantharidin, cryotherapy, electrocautery, radiocautery ablation, infrared coagulation, photodynamic therapy, and lasers.

4.1.1 Surgery

Curettage followed by cautery was an early and still widely practiced method of surgical removal of warts. A success rate of 65–85% has been reported in surgical therapy, but scarring and recurrence rate are high (30%), and the sole of the foot is the site where scarring is particularly problematic. Curettage followed by cautery is most commonly used for filiform warts on the limbs and face [8]. Excision is usually to be avoided as scarring is inevitable, and there is frequent chance of recurrence in the scar.

4.2 Salicylic acid

It is keratolytic, reduces the thickness of warts and may also stimulate an inflammatory response. Over-the-counter preparations are available as 17% salicylic acid combined in a base of flexible collodion or as a 40% salicylic acid plaster patch [9]. It is minimally expensive, convenient and reasonably effective, with negligible pain, but results require weeks to months of treatment. Occasionally, contact dermatitis due to colophony may develop, and to avoid systemic toxicity, it should be applied only in limited area. Treatment result with salicylic acid therapy extremely depends on patient compliance. Before pairing or debridement of the dead, hyperkeratotic tissue, wart(s) should be soaked in warm water for 5 min. The salicylic acid preparation should then be applied to the debrided wart [10].

4.3 Chemical cautery

Strong chemicals can destroy tissue. Trichloroacetic acid (**TCA**) and bichloroacetic acid (**BCA**) are not readily absorbed by tissue; it kills warts by denaturing and destroying the proteins in the cells. Treatment via **chemical cautery** with a solution of 60–90% trichloroacetic acid (TCA) is most effective when treating few small, moist lesions. There is a complete clearance of warts in 70% of patients who received up to 6 treatments of trichloroacetic acid. Thirty percent of patients who were treated with trichloroacetic acid developed ulcerations at the site of its application [11]. Recurrence rate is not clear. Silver nitrate is probably most widely recognised in its historical use to prevent conjunctivitis in newborns [12]. This treatment for warts is currently more widely used in the United Kingdom where non-prescription 95% silver nitrate caustic applicator pencils are available [13]. Chances of excessive burn and pigmentation are there.

4.4 Cantharidin

A terpenoid secreted by blister beetles, which is absorbed by lipids in keratinocytes, activates serine proteases and leads to acantholysis [14, 15]. Depending on the amount, concentration, duration of exposure and occlusion, an intraepidermal blister will form and resolve, within a week [16]. The superficial nature of the injury reduces the risk of scarring. One randomised control trial shows that cantharidin is effective, is safe, yields better cosmesis and requires fewer applications than TCA for the treatment of warts when used sufficiently far from mucosal and intertriginous areas. It was also shown to be well tolerated and that patients being treated with Cantharone were significantly more satisfied than those treated with TCA. This may be attributed to less pain during application and during the entire treatment, better cosmetic results and perhaps fewer visits [17].

4.5 Phenol (carbolic acid)

It is a strong caustic agent that can penetrate deep into tissue, produces chemical burn with escher and is not used routinely for treatment of common wart.

Strong (80%) phenol solution for the treatment of common warts showed that phenol was an effective form of treatment for warts. It must be used by a physician and should not be used in extensive areas [18].

4.6 Retinoic acid

Topical tretinoin, although currently recommended for the treatment of acne, has also been reported to be of benefit in plane warts. A study of 25 children with plane warts treated with 0.05% topical tretinoin cream (applied once daily for 6 weeks) was compared with a control group of 25 untreated children. After 12 weeks, clearance of warts was observed in 84.6% of the treated group as compared with 32% of the control group. It was well tolerated with some redness and peeling in 42.3% of the treated group [19].

4.7 Photodynamic therapy

Photodynamic therapy (PDT) with topical 5-aminolevulinic acid has a good curative effect, especially in recalcitrant facial flat warts [20–22]. It is unclear, but selective photothermolysis of oxyhaemoglobin within the dilated microvasculature of the warts leads to destruction of capillaries followed by improvement of warts, may be the mechanism of action of this curative effect [23]. Many factors affect the efficacy of PDT, including photosensitizer concentration; solvent type; incubation time; type, dose, and time of irradiation of the light; and the area of exposed parts. ALA gel (10%) was applied topically to lesions and incubated for 3 h. The lesions were irradiated by an LED light of 630 ± 10 nm at dose levels of 60–100 mW/cm. At the 24-week follow-up, the average effective rate was 88.8%, with no recurrences. No significant side effects were reported [24].

4.8 Cryotherapy

Cryotherapy induces cold thermal injury in the lesion. Cryotherapy may have an effect on wart clearance either by simple necrotic destruction of HPV-infected keratinocytes or possibly by inducing local inflammation conducive to the development of an effective cell-mediated response [25]. Dimethyl ether spray, carbon dioxide snow and liquid nitrogen all produce cold thermal damage to the skin. Different types of devices and techniques are used to induce targeted cold injury to warts. Carbon dioxide slush (−79°C) is now less commonly used.

4.8.1 Mixture of dimethyl ether and propane (DMEP)

It is in aerosol form, easy to handle and stored in normal room temperature, and its preservation time is very high (nearly 3 years), available in market and easy to buy. As the evaporation temperature reaches −57°, therefore, it is likely to be less effective, and efficacy in inducing tissue temperatures adequate for cell necrosis appears low [26]. But one multicentre RCT on comparing effects of DMEP and LN_2 shows that no clinically relevant differences between the efficacy, tolerance and safety of the two cryogenic agents used in primary care were found. The low freezing of DMEP was sufficient for the cryotherapy of benign lesions [27].

4.8.2 Liquid nitrogen therapy

Having a temperature of −196°C, the coldest freeze, is the most commonly used method in medical practice. It is very effective in elimination of a large variety of very common benign and premalignant skin lesions (verrucas, *Molluscum contagiosum*, seborrheic and actinic keratoses) [25]. Wart clearance may be through necrotic destruction of HPV-infected keratinocytes or by inducing local inflammation that triggers an effective cell-mediated response [25]. Liquid nitrogen can easily be stored and used by simple equipment in clinic-based practice. Available techniques are dipstick, roller, spray gun and Probe. Dipstick is the simplest technique where a cotton swab is dipped in liquid nitrogen and applied on a lesion. It is suitable only for superficial, benign lesions. Cryoroller, whose tip is cylindrical, is dipped in liquid nitrogen and then rolled over the lesional area. It acts better in severe acne and hypertrophic scar. The most popular method is spray technique using cryoprobes [10]. There are variations in freeze times, mode of application and intervals between treatments. Freeze time is the time elapsed from start to end of freeze cycle, i.e., from formation of uniform ice field until lesion is thawed, varying from 5 to 20 s. In short freeze for warts, cryotherapy continued till a 2-mm white halo develops around the lesion; this is enough for plane wart or filiform warts. But long freeze time (maintaining white halo for 5–20 s) is required for plantar warts. The cycle is repeated every 3 weeks on 8–10 occasions. It is better to pare hyperkeratotic lesions before cryosurgery as it acts as insulator. A cure rate of 60–80% can be anticipated [28]. Longer freeze is more effective than traditional (shorter) freeze, and blistering is significantly greater [29]. Plantar warts need comparatively more aggressive therapy. There is no difference between single freeze-thaw cycle and double freeze-thaw cycle in palmer warts but in plantar warts, and double freeze-thaw is more effective [30]. The number of session is important, not the interval between sessions for percentage cure [31]. Two-week intervals between sessions may be an optimal treatment [31].

4.9 Ablation radiofrequency

Localised heating with radiofrequency heat generators and surgical excision with radiofrequency electrosurgical knives have been used with moderate success [32, 33].

Radiofrequency ablation is a common mode of treatment, and it involves the principle of tissue destruction with various waveforms of alternating electric current whose frequencies fall within the range of radiofrequency (500–4000 khz) [34]. The overall cure rate for warts with radiosurgery ranges between 33 and 80% depending on the number of sittings and the type of warts [35, 36].

Electrocautery is a form of electrosurgery that utilises galvanic or direct current for generating heat. Although rarely used nowadays in the developed nations, it is still widely used in the developing countries and is considered more effective for treating thicker lesions with an overall success rate of 56–80% [7].

4.10 Infrared coagulation

It is an instrument that produces noncoherent infrared light with a spectrum of 400–2700 nm. It has been reported as a cheaper, safer and more easily handled alternative to CO_2 laser treatment. Direct application of infrared contact coagulators causes thermal injury to a depth dependent on the duration of exposure [37]. A bulla arises after IRC that may protect the lesion against infection. Cure rate was 66.7% for warts treated with IRC. The instrument allows adjustable tissue necrosis without tissue adhesion and has yielded remissions with a 10.8% recurrence rate [38]. In comparison to electrocoagulation, infrared coagulation produces similar outcomes [37], but it is safer than EC in side effect profile.

4.11 Laser therapy

4.11.1 Carbon dioxide (CO_2) laser

The CO_2 laser was the initial laser modality used to treat warts and has been used since 1980s [39–41]. The CO_2 laser emits infrared light of wavelength 10,600 nm. It is absorbed by tissue water and results nonselective thermal tissue destruction. The CO_2 laser treats warts via two mechanisms. A focused CO_2 laser beam used as a scalpel to excise the wart down to the subcutaneous tissue, followed by the base of the wart, which is vaporised by a defocused beam until a clean surgical field is obtained [42–45]. Cohort studies report that simple and recalcitrant common, palmar, plantar, periungual and subungual warts have been successfully treated with CO_2 laser, with response rates ranging from 50 to 100% [40, 43, 46–53]. Usually, excision by focused mode followed by vaporisation and haemostasis with defocused mode is the common practice. Deeper warts need more passes. Using two to four passes per wart is adequate [46–49]. CO_2 laser treatment may be used for recalcitrant warts but also as a first-line of therapy for warts—mainly in the sole, hands and other parts also [46]. Single verruca lesions usually result better (66.7%) than multiple verruca (62.5%) [46]. It can be used for first-line therapy for periungual and subungual warts. It has been seen that patients with subungual and periungual warts, who have failed previous conventional therapy, respond less than in patients when CO_2 laser therapy was given as first line (47.9% compared to 80.0%) [47]. Subungual warts respond better than periungual warts [47]. Usually one or two sessions are adequate [48]. Patients with one session heal earlier than patients with more than one session [48]. Adverse effects include permanent nail matrix damage and scarring, and nail changes such as distal onycholysis and thickening may occur [47, 48, 51]. CO_2 laser may also be used as excision tool, with a remission rate of 95.5%, but requires specialised unit [49]. Scarring is a possibility [49]. 'En bloc' excision of wart is very much effective [100%] in paediatric age group also with no recurrence, and usually single session is adequate [50]. Many treatment modalities are not feasible in immunosuppressive patients. CO_2 laser can be a safe and comparably effective modality of treatment, even in one intervention [51]. Complete excision of the lesional skin with a portion of deeper tissue and 1-mm non-lesional margin leads to the complete clearance of HPV DNA, which leads to very lower recurrence, though chance of scar formation is there. Dressing with artificial dermis leads to less scar formation [52]. Application of Imiquad after CO_2 laser in recalcitrant wart reduces or stops recurrences [53]. Vapour produced by CO_2 laser with any power density and fluence contains intact papillomavirus DNA. This infected vapour may cause pulmonary infection [54]. Plume produced from laser procedure collected and used as inoculum may produce identical lesions [55]. So, safety precautions during laser surgery may be strictly maintained [55]. It is important to wear surgical masks as it is capable of removing all laser- or electrocoagulation-derived viruses [56], even gas scavenging system to be in use [57]. But a study among CO_2 laser surgeons in all the members of American Society of Laser Medicine shows that the plume does not possess enough infectious material to produce significantly more amount of warts in laser surgeons in comparison to population-based common subjects [58]. But, sitewise, CO_2 laser surgeons have a greater risk of acquiring nasopharyngeal lesions, especially when they treat genital warts with HPV types 6 and 11 [58]. Scar formation is a known side effect of CO_2 lasers, and there are more chances of hypertrophic scar formation if the patient is on cyclosporine for other reasons [59]. In superpulsed CO_2 LASERs, the high irradiances and brief duration make possible very precise removal of target lesion volumes and controlled excision. Here, thermal damage is very less leading to less inflammation and less scarring [60].

4.11.2 Erbium:yttrium/aluminium/garnet (Er:YAG) laser

Non-ablative lasers are largely replacing ablative CO_2 lasers as side effects are less, both for patients and clinicians [61]. Er:YAG laser emits 2940 nm wavelength. It is absorbed 12–18 times more efficiently by water containing superficial cutaneous tissue than CO_2 laser. At 250 microsecond pulse duration and 5 J/cm^2 fluence short pulse, Er:YAG laser ablates 5–20 micrometre of tissue per laser pass, and minimal residual thermal damage that results faster tissue re-epithelialization and less side effects. The disadvantage is intraoperative bleeding [62]. Its mechanism of action in treating warts is through direct ablation of the lesion in the epidermis, layer by layer until normal tissue is visualised. This laser type also has bactericidal effects [61]. Er:YAG laser was tried in all types of common warts—periungual, subungual and plantar warts; complete clearance rate was 68% for plantar warts, 78% for periungual warts and 76% for subungual warts. In patients with extensive involvement, more than one session were needed. Relapse was only in plantar wart patients (17.8%) [62]. Chance of scarring is less in Er:YAG laser [62, 63]. For hard-to-treat palmoplantar warts, a combination of ablative Er:YAG laser and topical 0.5% podophyllotoxin solution yields higher success with complete clearance of 88.6% without any pigmentary changes, wound infection and scarring. Relapse rate is also less [64]. Er:YAG laser procedure can be done without anaesthesia or with topical cream anaesthesia as there is minimal pain, except only in large, very thick plaque in the plantar or palm. The plume contains no viral DNA [65]. Side effects are less with Er:YAG laser, no hyper- or hypopigmentation and no post-operative infection. Healing is very fast, within 7–10 days. Redness persists up to 3 months [66]. In a study of 69 patients with difficult-to-treat warts (periungual or plantar), 72.5% of patients with wart observed complete response (CR) irrespective of the duration of infection with HPV or the age of the patients. Plantar warts were more resistant (13.5% non-responders) than periungual warts (5.9% non-responders), and larger mosaic plantar warts were less sensitive than single warts; 24.0% of patients showed relapse [67]. Wound healing may be assisted/accelerated with LED phototherapy (633 nm). Immediately after Er:YAG ablation, with precise removal of wart tissue, a red LED therapy system is applied (633 nm, 20 min, 96 J/cm^2) to the wound and surrounding area, LED system with same parameters were repeated on the second, sixth and tenth post-operative day. On the sixth post-operative day, the wound has shrunk noticeably and is filled with healthy, granulation tissue, and on day 15, the wound healed completely with minimal scarring; recurrence rate was also less (<6%) [68].

4.11.3 Neodymium:YAG (Nd:YAG) laser

Principal emission of Nd:YAG is at 1064 nm, in the infrared range [Nd:YAG produces heat]. Heat therapy depends on the principle that diseased tissue which is being treated is more sensitive to the effects of the elevated temperature than normal tissue and this is less able to recover after heat exposure [69]. Side effects such as coagulation, blister or crusts are less after hyperthermia. Response is excellent (77%), though in 23% of the method failed, and there is no recurrence in 9 months follow-up. Nd:YAG can be used in all types and site warts including periungual, hand and plantar warts [70]. HPV DNA becomes completely absent in hyperthermia-treated wart lesions, in comparison to cryotherapy where 96% wart lesions are positive for HPV DNA by in situ hybridization [71]. The light of the solid state Nd:YAG laser can easily be guided by fibres to tissue and perform good coagulation and homeostatic function, in laryngeal, as well as genital, easily and more precisely. Its continuous suction endures a minimal load of potential infectious laser plume [72]. For therapeutic treatment, Nd:YAG laser can be utilised for genital tract lesion and cervical conization for early neoplasms like dysplasia, carcinoma in situ and microinvasive carcinoma [73, 74]; these are caused by HPV infections. Invasive lasers like CO_2 are normally considerably more painful and require longer recovery time, and also side effects like scarring are high. A long pulsed Nd:YAG laser emits 1064 nm wavelength light, in infrared spectrum, in longer wavelength with lower haemoglobin, and melanin absorption coefficients allows deeper delivery of higher energy in hyperkeratotic and thicker epidermis that are assisted with warts [75]. Several studies have evaluated the use of the Nd:YAG laser in the treatment of simple and recalcitrant common, palmoplantar, periungual and subungual warts, with efficacies ranging from 46 to 100% [61, 76–78]. Laser protocol varied among different studies: spot size between 3 and 7 mm, pulse duration of 1–20 ms, fluence of 100–200 J/cm^2, cooling methods, number of pulses between 1 and 8, treatment interval from 2 weeks to 12 months and mean number of treatments between 1.49 and 4.65. In a study of Han et al. [76], 348 patients of all types of simple and recalcitrant common, palmoplantar and periungual warts are treated with Nd:YAG laser (spot size, 5 mm; pulse duration, 20 ms; 200 J/cm^2; no cooling; 1–2 pulses). After a mean of 1.49 treatments, wart clearance rate was 96% though there were differences in clearance rates after initial treatment depending on location (72.6% for common warts vs. 44.1% for palmoplantar warts) [76]. For determination of effectiveness and safety of a novel 100 microsecond pulsed 1064 nm Nd:YAG laser in treatment of Verruca vulgaris, low energy (200 mjouls) Nd:YAG, in monthly intervals for 3 months was given to 25 patients with lesion on hands-nineteen patients had complete clearance; with minimal discomfort [61]. At least partial response (50% reduction) in verruca size was noticed in all lesions [61]. Aggressive treatment of hand warts may cause tissue damage. To avoid the tissue damage, a novel modification was tried [77]. Fifty one recalcitrant verrucas were treated with ND:YAG laser; all warts were administered in at least three pulses. The circle of pulses given in that way that the three circles overlapped each other only on the site of verruca- so that highest level of energy reached only to the wart. The adjacent tissue can avoid unintended tissue damage [77]. All lesions subsided, 88.35% lesions in one laser session, remaining patients were required two laser sessions- those lesions were periungual and palmar. There was no recurrence in 12 months follow-up, no major side effects, no nail dystrophy or severe post-treatment scarring. Hyperpigmentation was present in 5.48% patients [77].

4.11.4 Pulsed dye laser

Among non-ablative modalities, pulsed dye laser (PDL) can be used for a selective, non-bloody destruction of extragenital and genital warts [79]. It emits a wavelength of 585, which is absorbed by haemoglobin and oxyhaemoglobin [79, 80]. Mechanism of action is unclear, but may be a result of intense heating of dermal vessels that leads to damage of viral DNA-containing keratinocytes. The theory is based on the presence of dilated and congested vessels at the base of most verruca and the mechanism of selective photothermolysis that results in the targeting of haemoglobin by the PDL [80]. The heat and immunological process and the removal of the blood supply to the wart may be the reason for the effectiveness of PDL in verruca therapy, but it is not above controversy [81]. This selective damage to blood vessels, sparing unnecessary damage to healthy adjacent cellular structure, avoids the scarring [82]. The local dermal vascular destruction of the warts stimulates cell-mediated immune response that is important for eradication of viral warts [83]. So, PDL for wart therapy, even in facial wart, is attractive [84] for its efficient and cosmetic resolution [84, 85]. The PDL is usually painless or minimally painful like snapped by a rubber band [86], though some patients complain of severe intraoperative pain [87, 88], so local anaesthesia may be required. Purpura may develop due to sudden burst of wart vasculature—that develops within minutes in the treated areas—which takes 10–14 days to subside spontaneously [88]. Even perianal warts in child patients are also treatable with PDL without any complications and with 100% clearance [89]. Verruca plana lesions on face in Asian (type IV-V skin) clear completely with PDL without producing significant pigmentary and textural complications [90]. Safety is one of the major advantages of this technique [91]. But the absence of any proven superiority over the standard treatments in terms of efficacy, coupled with high costs, means that PDL should only be used as second-line therapy in patients with cosmetic needs [91].

Laser protocols are different in all studies, and variation of results may be for that reason. Different protocols include spot size of 5–10 mm, fluence of 5 j/m^2–15 j/m^2, pulse duration of 38 ns–1.5 ms, consecutive 2–3 pulses with overlap of 1–2 mm, 1–12 sessions, interval of 2–4 weeks and cooling methods [90–98]. In immunocompetent children, the overall response rate is 75%, and the remaining 25% had partial clearance, with an average number of treatment for complete clearance to be 3.1—face and perineum are areas most likely to be cleared in one treatment (50 and 20%, respectively) [99, 100]. It is also a more effective therapy especially against those that have not been eradicated by other treatments [101]. Though less, adverse effects are also not very much uncommon, about 8.2% of patients had adverse effects like wound formation (3.8%), residual scarring (2.9%), infection (1.0%) and collapse (0.5%); 63% of patients had excessive pain [97]. But opinion about pain and patient compliance are different in other study [102]. Here only 6.34% of patients classified the method as too painful and withdrew after the first one or two treatments They have concluded that FPDL is safe and effective for the removal or reduction of verrucae vulgares, and requires less patient compliance compared with other treatment options. PDL followed by intralesional Bleomycin gives very good result with complete clearance, even in immunosuppressive patients, though the overall treatment session was high (1.8 vs. 3) [98], but should be aware of common side effects seen such as painful haemorrhagic blistering and superficial ulceration [103].

4.11.5 Potassium titanyl phosphate (KTP) laser

The KTP laser has been utilised in the treatment of recalcitrant cutaneous warts, and when treated to complete clearance, no recurrence occurred [104].

5. Virucidal therapy

5.1 Glutaraldehyde

Glutaraldehyde is a tissue fixative that polymerises keratin. Its effectiveness lies in desiccation of surface virions and resultant reduction of antigenic load [105]. However the mechanism of action of glutaraldehyde against warts has not been clarified precisely. Glutaraldehyde therapy (GA) for warts was first introduced in 1971 [106]. Therapeutic responses with glutaraldehyde in periungual, palmar and plantar warts were 80, 60 and 68.5%, respectively [107]. When GA is buffered by suitable alkalinating agents to a pH of 7.5–8.5, the solution becomes antimicrobially active [108]. The concentration of glutaraldehyde is another consideration for use. Though 2 w/v% is the minimum for antimicrobial activity [108], undiluted high concentration of 25% solution appeared to work faster on warts of all kinds [107]. The benefits of using glutaraldehyde as first-line treatment for warts, especially resistant ones, are the same as those of cryotherapy [107].

5.2 Formaldehyde

Formalin (formaldehyde) is a virucidal agent and has strong disinfectant properties and exerts its effects by causing damage to the upper layers of epidermal cells that contain the virus, thus destroying viruses [28, 109]. Formalin application was effective in 83.3% of patients, but complete disappearance of warts was seen in 11.1% [110]. The most common side effects of formalin include redness, irritation and dryness of skin [111].

5.3 Acyclovir, valacyclovir and other antiretroviral drugs

Oral antivirals are not a regular treatment modality, but isolated case report about improvement in wart lesion after oral treatment with acyclovir [112], valacyclovir are there. Plantar wart is cleared completely with 1 gm valacyclovir for 60 days [113]. Improvements of wart with intravenous cidofovir in one HIV seropositive patient with complete clearance are available [114]. Nearly total clearance of multiple viral wart with didanosine, stavudine and efavirenz triple antiretroviral therapy in a 34-year-old male homosexual patient was seen, accompanied by a significant improvement in immune status [115]. The observations are not powerful enough to assume causality (instead of a simple casual or placebo effect).

6. Antimitotic therapy

6.1 Bleomycin

Bleomycin is a chemotherapeutic agent which has an antitumor, antibacterial and antiviral activity which may be related to its ability to bind with deoxyribonucleic acid (DNA), causing bleomycin strand scission and elimination of pyrimidine and purine bases [116]. It selectively affects squamous cell and reticuloendothelial tissue [117]. Bleomycin is not thought to bind directly to HPV [10]. Bleomycin causes acute tissue necrosis that may stimulate an immune response, as evidenced by the fact that it is less effective as a wart treatment in immunosuppressed renal transplant patients [118–121].

Adverse effects include injection pain and burning, erythema, swelling and pain within 24–72 h after injection before a black thrombotic eschar forms. Local complications after periungual injections are nail loss [122] or dystrophy [123]. Reynaud's phenomenon in treated fingers, local pigmentation [124] or urticaria [122], even flagellate hyperpigmentation [125] are reported after.

In a systemic review [126], comparing intralesional bleomycin with placebo, the studies have given conflicting results. Intralesional bleomycin was compared with saline or sesame oil; duration was 6 weeks to 3 months. The RCTs in the review favour I/L Bleomycin, and only one study opined placebo to be more effective. The result of wart clearance was between 18 and 94%, but the study showed clearance rate to be 94%, which was not significantly different from the result (73%) achieved by placebo injections of saline. Concentration of 0.5% bleomycin is more effective than concentration of 0.25% or 1% bleomycin. Pain was experienced by most patients, irrespective of doses. In a study of comparison between intralesional Bleomycin and cryotherapy, 0.1% concentration of bleomycin was used [127]. Greater efficacy in clearing warts was shown with intralesional bleomycin than in cryotherapy. The clearance rates of warts for intralesional bleomycin therapy found were 97%, and in 94.9% of patients, all warts treated with bleomycin were cleared. There was significantly less number of treatment sessions, with a mean of 1.38 in case of bleomycin treatment than the cryotherapy where the mean is 3.08.

6.2 Podophyllotoxin

Podophyllotoxin is a topical antimitotic that is purified from the plant families Coniferae and Berberidaceae (e.g. species of *Juniperus* and *Podophyllum*) or can be synthesised chemically. It is the active agent of podophyllin resin and is available as a 0.5% solution. Podophyllotoxin binds to microtubules and causes mitotic arrest in the metaphase of cell division [128]. Treatment should be limited to no more than 10 cm^2 of wart tissue, and no more than 0.5 mL/day of solution should be given. This is a patient-applied therapy. Podophyllin is a non-standardised unstable plant extract, derived from may apple (*Podophyllum peltatum Linné*), and contains the active agent podophyllotoxin. American *Podophyllum* contains one fourth the amount of podophyllotoxin than Indian *Podophyllum* does. The potency of podophyllin varies considerably between batches. The exact mechanism of action is unknown. Since it tends to work better on mucosal surfaces, it is used primarily to treat genital warts. Little information is available regarding treatment of non-genital warts with this medication. A single topical application of podophyllin cures less than one third of patients with genital warts [129, 130].

It results in necrosis when applied to anogenital warts. Only a trained medical professional can apply it, and it cannot be dispensed to a patient. CDC guidelines for anogenital warts, recommended regimens for External Anogenital Warts (i.e. penis, groin, scrotum, vulva, perineum, external anus and perianus), includes patient-applied therapy with podofilox (podophyllotoxin) 0.5% solution or gel—using a cotton swab or finger. This podofilox solution (using a cotton swab) or gel (using a finger) should be applied to anogenital warts twice daily for 3 consecutive days, followed by 4 days of drug interval. If necessary, it can be repeated, for up to four cycles. The total treated area should not exceed 10 cm^2, and up to 0.5 ml podofilox should be used per day [131]. If possible initial application should be demonstrated by one healthcare provider for demonstration of proper application and technique and to identify the appropriate warts for treatment. Mild to moderate pain or local irritation might develop after treatment [131].

Podophyllotoxin, the active ingredients of podophyllin, is contraindicated in pregnancy. Though human data not available during application in lactating mother, it is considered as potential toxic. Podophylline, a raw form, is also contraindicated in pregnancy and breastfeeding mother, due to the potential severe myelotoxicity and neurotoxicity in the mother, though no human data available. The American college of Obstetricians and Gynecologists and other sources contraindicated the use of podophyllum agents include the use of podophyllotoxin (podofilox) during pregnancy and in the vagina or cervix at any time [132]. In a randomised comparative study, 60 women with genital warts were treated with either weekly application of 20% podophyllin solution or self-treatment with 0.5% podophyllotoxin cream twice daily for 3 days in weekly intervals. Patients were treated for a maximum of four treatment cycles, and final assessment was carried out after 3 months. Podophyllotoxin cream had a significantly better clearance than podophyllin solution, a primary clearance of was 82% vs 59%. These final clearance decreased to 71% and 48% at the 3-month follow-up, respectively. Total wart clearance was 94% with podophyllotoxin and 74% with podophyllin solution. Podophyllin cream came to as easy to apply and effects significantly better than podophyllin solution. Local side effects were mild to moderate with erythema, and erosion appeared to be higher in the podophyllotoxin group but not so serious to discontinue treatment [133].

7. Immunotherapy

This treatment uses the patient's own immune system to fight the warts. Some types of immunotherapy only target certain cells of the immune system. Others affect the immune system in general. Because of the cumbersome nature of the conventional procedures and a high risk of recurrence, immunotherapy is becoming more and more popular, especially in the treatment of refractory cutaneous and genital warts. These include various topical, intralesional and systemic agents. There are no well-defined criteria or consensus on when immunotherapy should be tried in a patient with warts. Current indications [134] include the following (**Table 1**).

1. Recalcitrant warts

2. Recurrent warts

3. Extensive warts

4. Difficult-to-treat areas—periungual and palmoplantar sites

7.1 Imiquimod

Imiquimod is a non-nucleoside heterocyclic amine which acts as an immune response modifier that may stimulate cytokines, including interferon-α, interleukin-1, interleukin-6, tumour necrosis factor-α, granulocyte-macrophage colony-stimulating factor and granulocyte colony-stimulating factor [135]. In a quantitative systemic review of published randomised control trials, six RCTs were evaluated, and all six studies were conducted in the sitting of home administration

Agents	Indication, dosage and administration
Topical agents	
Imiquimod	For genital and cutaneous warts, 5% cream, 3 times a week, for 16 week
Sinecatechins	For cutaneous warts, 10% ointment 3 times a day for maximum 16 weeks
BCG	For cutaneous and genital warts, applied topically on the warts in normal saline or salicylic acid, washed after 2 hours, weekly treatment for 6 to 12 weeks
Intralesional (IL) agents	
Mw vaccine	For cutaneous warts, 0.1 ml intradermal into 3-5 warts or all warts, followed by 0.1 ml intralesional, 2-4 weekly, maximum 10 sittings
BCG vaccine	For cutaneous and genital warts, 0.1-0.5 ml intralesional injection in largest wart, in 2 weeks interval in 5 sittings.
PPD	For genital warts, 0.1 ml weekly intradermal injection in the forearm for 12 weeks
MMR vaccine	For cutaneous warts, 0.3-0.5 ml into single largest wart fortnightly for up to 5 sittings
Candidial extract	For cutaneous warts, 0.1-0.3 ml injected into the largest wart at first sitting, then 3 weekly intralesional injections
Trichophyton antigen	For cutaneous and genital warts, 0.3 ml injected into largest wart every 3 weeks, maximum of 5 sittings
Tuberculin	For cutaneous warts, 2.5 units into few warts every 2 weekly
Vitamin D3	For cutaneous warts, 0.2 ml of 7.5 mg/ml, Vitamin D intralesional, 2 sittings 4 week apart
Interferon alpha 2B	For genital warts, 1-2 million units 3 days/week (Monday-Wednesday-Friday) for 3 weeks
Systemic	
Zinc	For cutaneous warts, 10mg/kg/day (2.5 mg/kg/day elemental zinc) for 2 months
Cimetidine	For cutaneous warts, 20-40 mg/kg/day for 3-4 months
Levamisole	For cutaneous warts, 2.5-5 mg/kg/day, 2-3 consecutive days every 2 weeks for 4-5 months.
Echinacea	For cutaneous warts, 600 mg single oral dose (single study)
Propolis	For cutaneous warts, 500 mg single oral dose (single study)
HPV vaccines	For cutaneous warts, 0.5 ml intramuscularly, at 0, 2 and 6 months (2 dose or 3 dose regimen) may be followed

Courtesy of Prof Devinder M Thappa and Minu J Chiramel [134].

Table 1.
Various agents used in immunotherapy of warts.

after initial professional examination and advice wart locations are genital, both in males and females. Five of the studies are on immunocompetent patients and one study on HIV-positive patients; 90% of the study population are male. Imiquimod was used as 5% cream in 4 trials and 2% cream in one trial, with complete clearance achieved in 51% in imiquimod group but only 6% patients in placebo group. The number needed to treat (NNT) was 2.2 (95% confidence interval 2.0–2.6). At least 50% reduction in wart area occurred in 72% of patients treated with Imiquimod 5% cream and 20% in placebo treated group. The number needed to treat was 1.9 (1.7–2.2). Warts were completely cured and did not recur in 37% (31% to 43%) of patients treated with imiquimod 5%, and 4% (2% to 6%) of patients treated with placebo. The NNT was 3.0 (2.5 to 3.8). Fewer patients were cured with 1% imiquimod in two trials, and for this concentration the NNT was 9.5 (5.9 to 25). Imiquimod 5% cream was significantly more effective than imiquimod 1% cream for complete wart clearance [136]. Common adverse events were localised itching, erythema, burning and erosion or excoriation, there was rarely any withdrawal from study due to these adverse effects. In HIV infected patients with warts, at least 50% reduction of wart area was seen in 38%, and in placebo it was 14%. Adverse events were similar to non-HIV group [137]. It is found to be effective and safe in children and there are reports of safe use in pregnancy [138, 139]. Disadvantages of using imiquimod 5% cream were the high cost and the length of average treatment (9.5 weeks).

7.2 *Mycobacterium w*

Mycobacterium indicus pranii or *Mycobacterium w* is rapid growing nontubercular mycobacteria, which has been found to induce a strong pro-inflammatory response while injected intralesionally. There is a prominent delayed hypersensitivity response, leading to clearance of warts both at the site of injection and distally [140]. The response varied by 54–93% in cutaneous warts and 89% in genital warts [140–143]. It is administered in two ways—either with an intradermal sensitising dose or without it. In the first method, a sensitising dose of 0.1 ml is administered intradermally in the deltoid region followed by 2–4 weekly intralesional injections in few warts (maximum 0.1 ml in each sitting) for up to 10 sittings. In the latter, the sensitization dose is missed, and direct intralesional injections are started [140, 141]. Mycobacterium *w* vaccine came as equally efficacious in treatment of refractory extragenital warts in comparison with cryotherapy and Imiquimod, 5%,. Mw vaccine has an added advantage of clearance of distant warts and reduction of viral load [144, 145]. The reported side effects include pain, nodularity, ulceration, scarring at the site of injection, flu-like symptoms, fever and lymphadenopathy [143]. Paraesthesia on the limb distal to the site of injection has also been reported [146].

7.3 *Bacillus* Calmette-Guérin vaccine

The delayed hypersensitivity response against the antigen is the key to clinical response against warts, same as that of the Mw vaccine. It increases the serum levels of IL-12 and decreases the level of IL-4 [147]. One to three doses are administered 1 month apart. In cutaneous warts (common, plantar, and plane warts), there was a resolution rate of 39.7% [148]. Topically applied BCG paste (weekly for 6 weeks) has also been found to be effective in children with common warts and plane warts with 65% resolution [149], and usually there are no side effects. However, another report in India showed a high incidence of flu-like symptoms precluding further doses in 57% of patients, making one question its safety in tuberculosis endemic countries like India [150].

7.4 MMR vaccine, *Candida, Trichophyton and tuberculin* antigens

Various types of vaccines and antigens were tried for wart management. Measles, mumps and rubella (MMR) viral vaccine accelerates the clearance of virus and viral infected cells by stimulation of cell-mediated and humoral immunity [151]. In this double-blind RCT, MMR vaccine was tried for three injections in 2-week interval with normal saline as control; 75% of patients had complete clearance, and another 16.6% had more than 50% clearance. There were no side effects, and in 6-month follow-up, there was no relapse [151]. In another study of MMR vaccine, 81.4% of patients had complete clearance; another 10% had partial clearance, in comparison to 27.5% and 15% with saline control [152]. A preliminary, open-label (PPD: purified protein derivative) study to investigate the effectiveness of the tuberculin antigen in the treatment of recalcitrant warts, taking advantage of the vaccination schedule in their country was designed. Three consecutive intralesional tuberculin (5TU PPD RT23-tween 80 solution) injections with 3-week intervals into each target wart, depending on the tuberculin reactivity, were performed. Injections of 0.3, 0.2 and 0.1 mL of antigen were administered to patients with indurations of 5–9, 10–15 and > 15 mm, respectively. Five patients (29.4%) demonstrated complete clearance, five (29.4%) had partial and five (29.4%) minimal response. Some patients showed complete clearance of untreated facial warts also. Patients with initial PPD test site in duration less than 10 mm had no or minimal response [153]. Mumps and *Candida* antigen injection in paediatric age group with recalcitrant warts had 47% complete resolution, and 13% had partial resolution. Injections were given in three weekly intervals, and an average of 3.87 injections was given. Patients with initial high response to skin antigen test shows excellent result [154]. Injection with mumps, *Candida* or *Trichophyton* antigen, alone or in combination, is given in 3-week interval, up to 10 injections. In patients who have completed the study, 50% had complete clearance, and the other 50% had 75–90% clearance. Local erythema and oedema were the only side effects, in 30% of patients. Patients who had complete clearance had clearance also in their distant verruca lesions [155]. *Candida albicans* intralesional immunotherapy in single also came as safe, well tolerated and suitable for multiple warts of hand and fingers, plantar warts and recalcitrant warts, even in non-injected warts [156]. In a randomised, single blinded, placebo-controlled large study of mumps, *Candida* and *Trichophyton* antigen, with or without interferon α 2b, 41% of patients with antigen alone, 57% antigen and interferon and 9% in only interferon had complete clearance in comparison to 19% only in the normal saline group [157]. The combination of mumps, *Candida* and *Trichophyton* also came to be effective as 74% of patients responded to test antigen had complete clearance with significant number also showing resolution of untreated distant warts [158]. Response of other studies with *Candida* antigen varied as 72% [159], 74% [160], 85% [161], 56% [162] and 87% [163], indicating antigen therapy in wart is a good hope for target and distant wart lesions with minimum side effects.

7.5 Interferons

Interferon has been shown to be active against HPV both in vitro and in vivo, to protect murine cells against infection with bovine papillomaviruses and to eliminate extrachromosomal viral DNA from infected cells [164, 165]. In a systematic meta-analysis, the rate of complete response in locally used interferon was 44.4% in comparison to placebo, 16.1%. The complete response rate of systemically used interferon as compared to placebo for treating genital warts had no perceivable discrepancy, for systemically used interferon 27.4% and placebo 26.4%. Both groups had near same recurrence rate (interferon 21.1% vs. placebo 34.2%, $p > 0.05$). In subgroup analysis, it was noticed that relapse was less in intralesional interferon in comparison to placebo group, but relapse rate were the same in between systemic and placebo groups. Adverse events were mostly mild and transient and could be tolerated [166].

7.6 Zinc

Dietary zinc has profound effects on the human immune system and deficiency leads to reduced immune capacity [167, 168]. It can be given as topical preparation, oral medication or intralesional. Topical preparation as 10% zinc sulphate lotion yields complete clearance in 80% in plane wart [169]; plane warts were seen in 85.7% [170]. Complete clearance noticed in 61% patients after 1 month therapy and 87% after 2 months of therapy with oral zinc sulphate 10 mg/kg/day in a placebo-controlled trial [171]. But it was not the same in other studies, 50% complete clearance with the same dose after 2 months in another open level clinical study [172]. Intralesional 2% zinc sulphate too has been found to induce clearance of warts [173].

7.7 H2 receptor blockers

H2 blockers, such as cimetidine and ranitidine, have been tried in treatment of warts. They block the type 2 histamine receptors on suppressor T cells and augment cell-mediated immunity [174]. It increases the levels of IFNγ and IL-2 and decreases the levels of IL-18 [175]. It has been used in a dose of 20–40 mg/kg/day for 3–4 months with response rate ranging from 30 to 87% [176, 177]. There is no significant difference between cimetidine and placebo [178], and some author proposed a placebo effect for cimetidine [179].

7.8 Levamisole

Levamisole, an antihelminthic agent, is found to have immunomodulatory effects, making it effective in various dermatological disorders including viral warts at a dose of 2.5–5 mg/kg/day for 3 consecutive days every 2 weeks for 4–5 months [180–182]. The response to levamisole was approximately 60%. Side effects are rash, nausea, abdominal cramps, taste alteration, alopecia, arthralgia and a flu-like syndrome and rarely cause myopathy, leukocytoclastic vasculitis, lichenoid eruptions and leukoencephalopathy [183, 184].

7.9 HPV vaccines

Since 2006, two vaccines against Human papillomavirus (HPV) have been licenced in more than 100 countries [185]. Both vaccines target HPV types 16 and 18, which account for about 70% of all cervical cancer cases, and the quadrivalent vaccine also targets HPV types 6 and 11, associated with 90% of genital warts (GWs) [186]. In Denmark, the quadrivalent HPV vaccine was introduced into the children's vaccination programme in January 2009 for 12-year-old girls. In 2014 the European Medicines Agency and the World Health Organisation Strategic Advisory Group of Experts recommended a two-dose schedule for 9–13-year-old girls. However, three-dose schedule offers better protection against genital warts than a two-dose schedule in a nationwide study. But, if the dosing interval extends (about six months), the two dose schedule came as effective as three. The quadrivalent HPV vaccine that comprises the L1 protein of HPV types 6, 11, 16 and 18 has been in use on a large scale in countries like Denmark with a decline in the prevalence of genital warts [187]. Similar decline in genital warts has been noticed in the UK and Australia [188, 189].

7.10 Autoimplantation therapy

Autowart inoculation by means of homologous autoimplantation helping to induce specific cell-mediated immunity has been proposed as a treatment option for recalcitrant, extensive and genital wart [190]. About 83 patients with all types of wart lesions were included in a study. At 16 weeks of therapy, 69.5% of patients recovered completely, and more than 75% improvement occurred in another 8.5% patients. No significant complication was documented. There was no recurrence within study period [191]. Another study also had noticed 73.3% total clearance of warts, with a majority of them (91%) within 2 months [190]. Inoculation site infection and post-inflammatory hyperpigmentation and hypopigmentation are the side effects.

7.11 Contact sensitizers

Contact sensitizers are a mode of inducing a type IV hypersensitivity reaction, thus making them a form of topical immunotherapy [28]. Diphencyprone (DCP) is the preferred compound. DCP 2% solution is applied after every 10–14 days, on the medial side of upper arm—till there is appearance of local erythema and vesiculation—and this may be repeated up to three times. Warts were then first pared followed by application with stepwise concentration of DCP: 0.01, 0.05, 0.10, 0.25, 0.50, 1.0, 1.5, 2.0, 3.0, 4.0 and 6.0%. Treatments are applied every 1–4 weeks. Resistant palmoplantar warts treated with DCP over 8 years [192] exhibited 88% clearance rate. However, a large percentage of patients developed adverse effects (56%), including painful blistering at the site of sensitization and near warts, pompholyx-like or generalised eczematous eruption, influenza-like symptoms, vesiculation elsewhere due to passive transfer of DCP and inguinal lymphadenopathy. They concluded that patients with recalcitrant palmar, plantar, periungual and digital warts are good candidates for DCP therapy [193].

8. Others

There are various other agents being tried infrequently in the management of warts.

Historic folk remedies have included many variants.

Duct tape occlusion therapy involves placing a piece of duct tape over the wart. The mechanism of action of this technique still remains unknown [194].

Components of garlic (*Allium sativum*) have been shown to have antiviral activity and to inhibit cellular proliferation of virally infected cells, resulting clearance of wart with less recurrence [195].

Application of paste made of baking powder and castor oil is age old technique for warts.

Herbal preparations such as Echinacea and propolis are reported to boost the immunity when administered orally [196], act as immunomodulators and improve warts.

Sinecatechins are derived from green tea extract (*Camellia sinensis*) and are marketed as a 10% ointment, containing around eight catechins. A clearance rate of 46–52% has been noticed in various studies [197].

Glycyrrhizic acid, obtained from the root of *Glycyrrhiza glabra*, has antiviral, anti-inflammatory and antiulcerative properties. When used with an immunostimulant [198], it was shown to have a slightly better efficacy than podophyllin (87%). The glycyrrhizic acid is a safe and effective treatment for the management of anogenital warts during pregnancy [199].

Intralesional injection of 0.2 ml of 15 mg/kg vitamin D3 led to complete resolution [200] in 19 (82.60%) out of 23 patients with palmoplantar warts and 14 (77.77%) of 18 patients with verruca vulgaris.

9. Conclusion

Numerous varieties of approaches for wart management are there. It is difficult to choose the best wart treatment. It should be determined by type of wart, whether old or new; site; immune status of the patient; pregnancy; the effects and side effects of the wart management procedure; its compliance with patient; and above all the availability of the planned modality of treatment. A rational consideration of all factors can provide an appreciable benefit.

Author details

Suchibrata Das
Department of Dermatology, Venereology and Leprosy, Nil Ratan Sircar Medical College, Kolkata, West Bengal, India

*Address all correspondence to: suchibratadas@yahoo.com

References

[1] Bzhalava D, Guan P, Franceschi S, Dillner J, Clifford G. A systematic review of the prevalence of mucosal and cutaneous human papillomavirus types. Virology. 2013;**445**:224-231

[2] Abeck D, Tetsch L, Lüftl M, Biedermann T. Extragenital cutaneous warts—Clinical presentation, diagnosis and treatment. Journal of the German Society of Dermatology. 2019;**17**(6):613-634

[3] Piaserico S, Sandini E, Pescerico A, et al. Cutaneous viral infections in organ transplant patients. Giornale Italiano di Dermatologia e Venereologia. 2014;**149**:409-415

[4] Maor D, Brennand S, Goh MSY, Chong AH. Recalcitrant hyperkeratotic verrucae in a renal transplant recipient clearing with cessation of immunosuppression. JAAD Case Reports. 2018;**24**:471-473

[5] Grassegger A, Rollinger-Holzinger I, Zelger BW, et al. Spontaneous or interferon-y induced T cell infiltration, HLA-DR and ICAM1 expression in genitoanal warts are associated with TH1 or mixed TH1/TH2 cytokine mRNA expression profiles. Archives of Dermatological Research. 1997;**289**:243-250

[6] Sterling JC, Gibbs S, Haque Hussain SS, Mohd Mustapa MF, Handfield-Jones SE. British Association of Dermatologists' guidelines for the management of cutaneous warts 2014. The British Journal of Dermatology. 2014;**171**(4):696-712. DOI: 10.1111/bjd.13310. Epub 2014 October 1

[7] Kuykendall-Ivy TD, Johnson SM. Evidence-based review of management of nongenital cutaneous warts. Cutis. 2003;**71**:213-222

[8] Lipke MM. An armamentarium of wart treatments. Clinical Medicine & Research. 2006;**4**(4):273-293

[9] Bedinghaus JM, Niedfeldt MW. Over-the-counter foot remedies. American Family Physician. 2001;**64**:791-796

[10] Baumbach JL, Sheth PB. Topical and intralesional antiviral agents. In: Wolverton S, editor. Comprehensive Dermatologic Drug Therapy. Philadelphia, PA: W. B. Saunders Company; 2001. pp. 524-536

[11] Abdullah AN, Walzman M, Wade A. Treatment of external genital warts comparing cryotherapy (liquid nitrogen) and trichloroacetic acid. Sexually Transmitted Diseases. 1993;**20**(6):344-345

[12] Hanif J, Tasca RA, Frosh A, Ghufoor K, Stirling R. Silver nitrate: Histological effects of cautery on epithelial surfaces with varying contact times. Clinical Otolaryngology and Allied Sciences. 2003;**28**:368-370

[13] Bray Healthcare. Silver Nitrate Pencil Instructions. Faringdon, Oxon, UK: Bray Group Ltd. Available at: http://www.bray.co.uk/silver-nitrate-pencil.html

[14] Haddad V Jr et al. Tropical dermatology: Venomous arthropods and human skin: Part I. Insecta. Journal of the American Academy of Dermatology. 2012;**67**(3):331.e1-331.14. [PubMed] [Google Scholar]

[15] Bertaux B et al. Cantharide acantholysis: Endogenous protease activation leading to desmosomal plaque dissolution. The British Journal of Dermatology. 1988;**118**(2):157-165. [PubMed] [Google Scholar]

[16] Torbeck R, Pan M, DeMoll E. Cantharidin: A comprehensive review

of the clinical literature. Dermatology Online Journal. 2014;**20**(6):3. [PubMed] [Google Scholar]

[17] Recanati MA, Kramer KJ, Maggio JJ, Chao CR. Cantharidin is superior to trichloroacetic acid for the treatment of non-mucosal genital warts: A pilot randomized controlled trial. Clinical and Experimental Obstetrics & Gynecology. 2018;**45**(3):383-386

[18] Banihashemi M, Pezeshkpoor F, Yazdanpanah MJ, Family S. Efficacy of 80% phenol solution in comparison with cryotherapy in the treatment of common warts of hands. Singapore Medical Journal. 2008;**49**(12):1035

[19] Kubeyinje EP. Evaluation of the efficacy and safety of 0.05% tretinoin cream in the treatment of plane warts in Arab children. Journal of Dermatological Treatment. 1996;**7**:21-22

[20] Mizuki D, Kaneko T, Hanada K. Successful treatment of topical photodynamic therapy using 5-aminolevulinic acid for plane warts. The British Journal of Dermatology. 2003;**149**:1087-1088

[21] Lin MY, Xiang LH. Topical 5-aminolevulinic acid photodynamic therapy for recalcitrant facial flat wart in Chinese subjects. The Journal of Dermatology. 2008;**35**:658-661

[22] Lu YG, Wu JJ, He Y, Yang HZ, Yang YD. Efficacy of topical aminolevulinic acid photodynamic therapy for the treatment of verruca planae. Photomedicine and Laser Surgery. 2010;**28**:561-563

[23] Morton CA, Szeimies RM, Sidoroff A, Braathen LR. European guidelines for topical photodynamic therapy part 2: Emerging indications—Field cancerization, photorejuvenation and inflammatory/infective dermatoses. Journal of the European Academy of Dermatology and Venereology. 2013;**27**:672-679

[24] Yang Y-l, Sang J, Liao N-x, Wei F, Liao W, Chen J-h. Off-label photodynamic therapy for recalcitrant facial flat warts using topical 5-aminolevulinic acid. Lasers in Medical Science. 2016 Jul;**31**(5):929-936. DOI: 10.1007/s10103-016-1925-8 Epub 2016 April 8

[25] Sterling JC, Handfield-Jones S, Hudson PM, British Association of Dermatologists. Guidelines for the management of cutaneous warts. The British Journal of Dermatology. 2001;**144**:4-11

[26] Gaspar ZS, Dawber RP. An organic refrigerant for cryosurgery: Fact or fiction? Australian Journal of Dermatology. 1997;**38**:71-72

[27] Caballero Martínez F et al. Dermatological cryosurgery in primary care with dimethyl ether propane spray in comparison with liquid nitrogen. Atencion Primaria. 1996;**18**(5):211-216

[28] Leman JA, Benton EC. Verrucas. Guidelines for management. American Journal of Clinical Dermatology. 2000;**1**:143-149

[29] Connolly M, Bazmi K, O'Connell M, Lyons JF, Bourke JF. Cryotherapy of viral warts: A sustained 10-s freeze is more effective than the traditional method. The British Journal of Dermatology. 2001;**145**:554-557

[30] Berth-Jones J, Bourke J, Eglitis H, Harper C, Kirk P, Pavord S, et al. Value of a second freeze-thaw cycle in cryotherapy of common warts. The British Journal of Dermatology. 1994;**131**:883-886

[31] Bourke JF, Berth-Jones J, Hutchinson PE. Cryotherapy of common viral warts at intervals of 1, 2 and 3 weeks. The British Journal of Dermatology. 1995;**132**:433-436

[32] Zaza M, Grassi C, Mardjonovic A, Valli E, Farne C, Romanini C. The use

of electrosurgery in the treatment of extra-cervical genital condylomatosis. Minerva Ginecologica. 1998;**50**:367-371

[33] Tosti A, Piraccini BM. Warts of the nail unit: Surgical and nonsurgical approaches. Dermatologic Surgery. 2001;**27**:235-239

[34] Wyre HW Jr, Stolar R. Extirpation of warts by a loop electrode and cutting current. The Journal of Dermatologic Surgery and Oncology. 1977;**3**:520-522

[35] Ferenczy A, Bergeron C, Richart RM. Human papillomavirus DNA in fomites on objects used for the management of patients with genital human papillomavirus infections. Obstetrics and Gynecology. 1989;**74**:950-954

[36] Dogra A, Gupta SK, Bansal A. Comparative efficacy of topical 5% FU with electrosurgey in treatment of warts. Indian Journal of Dermatology. 2006;**51**:108-110

[37] Piskin S, Aksoz T, Gorgulu A. The treatment of common warts with infrared coagulation. The Journal of Dermatology. 2004;**31**:989-992

[38] Bekassy Z, Westrom L. Infrared coagulation in the treatment of condyloma acuminata in the female genital tract. Sexually Transmitted Diseases. 1987;**14**:209-212

[39] Apfelberg DB, Druker D, Maser MR, White DN, Lash H, Spector P. Benefits of the CO_2 laser for verruca resistant to other modalities of treatment. The Journal of Dermatologic Surgery and Oncology. 1989;**15**(4):371-375

[40] Mancuso JE, Abramow SP, Dimichino BR, Landsman MJ. Carbon dioxide laser management of plantar verruca: A 6-year follow-up survey. The Journal of Foot Surgery. 1991;**30**(3):238-243

[41] McBurney EI, Rosen DA. Carbon dioxide laser treatment of verrucae vulgares. The Journal of Dermatologic Surgery and Oncology. 1984;**10**(1):45-48

[42] Serour F, Somekh E. Successful treatment of recalcitrant warts in pediatric patients with carbon dioxide laser. European Journal of Pediatric Surgery. 2003;**13**:219-223

[43] Logan RA, Zachary CB. Outcome of carbon dioxide laser therapy for persistent cutaneous viral warts. The British Journal of Dermatology. 1989;**121**(1):99-105

[44] Takac S. The CO_2 laser and verruca vulgaris [in Croatian]. Medicinski Pregled. 2000;**53**(7-8):389-393

[45] Hruza GJ. Laser treatment of warts and other epidermal and dermal lesions. Dermatologic Clinics. 1997;**15**(3):487-506

[46] Sloan K, Haberman H, Lynde CW. Carbon dioxide laser-treatment of resistant verrucae vulgaris: Retrospective analysis. Journal of Cutaneous Medicine and Surgery. 1998;**2**(3):142-145

[47] Lim JT, Goh CL. Carbon dioxide laser treatment of periungual and subungual viral warts. The Australasian Journal of Dermatology. 1992;**33**(2):87-91

[48] Street ML, Roenigk RK. Recalcitrant periungual verrucae: The role of carbon dioxide laser vaporization. Journal of the American Academy of Dermatology. 1990;**23**(1):115-120

[49] Oni G, Mahaffey PJ. Treatment of recalcitrant warts with the carbon dioxide laser using an excision technique. Journal of Cosmetic and Laser Therapy. 2011;**13**(5):231-236

[50] Serour F, Somekh E. Successful treatment of recalcitrant warts in

pediatric patients with carbon dioxide laser. European Journal of Pediatric Surgery. 2003;**13**(4):219-223

[51] Läuchli S, Kempf W, Dragieva G, Burg G, Hafner J. CO_2 laser treatment of warts in immunosuppressed patients. Dermatology. 2003;**206**(2):148-152

[52] Mitsuishi T, Sasagawa T, Kato T, et al. Combination of carbon dioxide laser therapy and artificial dermis application in plantar warts: Human papillomavirus DNA analysis after treatment. Dermatologic Surgery. 2010;**36**(9):1401-1405

[53] Zeng Y, Zheng YQ, Wang L. Vagarious successful treatment of recalcitrant warts in combination with CO_2 laser and imiquimod 5% cream. Journal of Cosmetic and Laser Therapy. 2014;**16**(6):311-313

[54] Garden JM, O'Banion MK, Shelnitz LS, Pinski KS, Bakus AD, Reichmann ME, et al. Papillomavirus in the vapor of carbon dioxide laser-treated verrucae. JAMA. 1988;**259**:1199-1202

[55] Garden JM, O'Banion MK, Bakus AD, Olson C. Viral disease transmitted by laser-generated plume (aerosol). Archives of Dermatology. 2002;**138**:1303-1307

[56] Sawchuk WS, Weber PJ, Lowy DR, Dzubow LM. Infectious papillomavirus in the vapor of warts treated with carbon dioxide laser or electrocoagulation: Detection and protection. Journal of the American Academy of Dermatology. 1989;**21**:41-49

[57] Kashima HK, Kessis T, Mounts P, Shah K. Polymerase chain reaction identification of human papillomavirus DNA in CO_2 laser plume from recurrent respiratory papillomatosis. Otolaryngology and Head and Neck Surgery. 1991;**104**:191-195

[58] Gloster HM Jr, Roenigk RK. Risk of acquiring human papillomavirus from the plume produced by the carbon dioxide laser in the treatment of warts. Journal of the American Academy of Dermatology. 1995;**32**:436-441

[59] Ozluer SM, Chuen BY, Barlow RJ, Markey AC. Hypertrophic scar formation following carbon dioxide laser ablation of plantar warts in cyclosporin-treated patients. The British Journal of Dermatology. 2001;**145**(6):1005-1007

[60] Hobbs ER, Bailin PL, Wheeland RG, Ratz JL. Superpulsed lasers: Minimizing thermal damage with short duration, high irradiance pulses. The Journal of Dermatologic Surgery and Oncology. 1987;**13**(9):955-964

[61] Goldberg DJ, Beckford AN, Mourin A. Verruca vulgaris: Novel treatment with a 1064 nm Nd:YAG laser. Journal of Cosmetic and Laser Therapy. 2015;**17**(2):116-119

[62] Wollina U. Erbium-YAG laser therapy—Analysis of more than 1200 treatments. Global Dermatology. 2016;**3**(2):268-272

[63] Park JH, Hwang ES, Kim SN, Kye YC. Er:YAG laser treatment of verrucous epidermal nevi. Dermatologic Surgery. 2004;**30**:378-381

[64] Wollina U. Er:YAG laser followed by topical podophyllotoxin for hard-to-treat palmoplantar warts. Journal of Cosmetic and Laser Therapy. 2003;**5**:35-37

[65] Hughes PS, Hughes AP. Absence of human papillomavirus DNA in the plume of erbium:YAG laser-treated warts. Journal of the American Academy of Dermatology. 1998;**38**:426-428

[66] Drnovšek-Olup B, Vedlin B. Use of Er:YAG laser for benign skin disorders.

Lasers in Surgery and Medicine. 1997;**21**(1):13-19

[67] Wollina U, Konrad H, Karamfilov T. Treatment of common warts and actinic keratoses by Er:YAG laser. Journal of Cutaneous Laser Therapy. 2001;**3**(2):63-66

[68] Trelles MA, Allones I, Mayo E. Er:YAG laser ablation of plantar verrucae with red LED therapy-assisted healing. Photomedicine and Laser Surgery. 2006;**24**(4):494-498

[69] Pfau A, Abd-el-Raheem TA, Baumler W, Hohenleutner U, Landthaler M. Nd:YAG laser hyperthermia in the treatment of recalcitrant verrucae vulgares (Regensburg's technique). Acta Dermato-Venereologica. 1994;**74**:212-214

[70] Pfau A, Abd-El-Raheem TA, Baumler W, Hohenleutner U, Landthaler M. Treatment of recalcitrant verrucae vulgares with Nd: YAG laser hyperthermia (Regensburg's technique): Preliminary results in 31 cases. Journal of Dermatological Treatment. 1995;**6**:39-42

[71] El-Tonsy MH, Anbar TE, El-Domyati M, Barakat M. Density of viral particles in pre and post Nd: YAG laser hyperthermia therapy and cryotherapy in plantar warts. International Journal of Dermatology. 1999;**38**:393-398

[72] Janda P, Leunig A, Sroka R, Betz CS, Rasp G. Preliminary report of endo-laryngeal and endotracheal laser surgery of juvenile-onset recurrent respiratory papillomatosis by Nd:YAG laser and a new fiber guidance instrument. Otolaryngology and Head and Neck Surgery. 2004;**131**:44-49

[73] Buzalov S, Khristakieva E. Condylomata acuminata. The correlation between affecting sexual partners and the risk of developing preneoplasia of the cervix uteri, The therapeutic potentials of the Nd-Yag laser. Akush Ginekol (Sofiia). 1999;**38**(3):36-38

[74] Izumi T, Kyushima N, Genda T, Kobayashi N, Kanai T, Wakita K, et al. Margin clearance and HPV infection do not influence the cure rates of early neoplasia of the uterine cervix by laser conization. European Journal of Gynaecological Oncology. 2000;**21**:251-254

[75] Kimura U, Takeuchi K, Kinoshita A, Takamori K, Suga Y. Long-pulsed 1064-nm neodymium:yttrium-aluminum-garnet laser treatment for refractory warts on hands and feet. The Journal of Dermatology. 2014;**41**(3):252-257

[76] Han TY, Lee JH, Lee CK, Ahn JY, Seo SJ, Hong CK. Long-pulsed Nd:YAG laser treatment of warts: Report on a series of 369 cases. Journal of Korean Medical Science. 2009;**24**(5):889-893

[77] Bingol UA, Comert A, Cinar C. The overlapped triple circle pulse technique with Nd:YAG laser for refractory hand warts. Photomedicine and Laser Surgery. 2015;**33**(6):338-342

[78] Baczako A, Krautheim V, Biedermann T, Volz T. Combination of surgery and Nd:YAG laser therapy for recalcitrant viral warts: A successful therapeutic approach for immunosuppressed patients. Acta Dermato-Venereologica. 2019;**99**:349-350

[79] El-Mohamady AE-S, Mearag I, El-Khalawany M, Elshahed A, Shokeir H, Mahmoud A. Pulsed dye laser versus Nd:YAG laser in the treatment of plantar warts: A comparative study. Lasers in Medical Science. 2014;**29**:1111-1116

[80] Robson KJ, Cunningham NM, Kruzan KL, et al. Pulsed-dye laser

versus conventional therapy in the treatment of warts: A prospective randomized trial. Journal of the American Academy of Dermatology. 2000;**43**(2, pt 1):275-280

[81] Schellhaas U, Gerber W, Hammes S, Ockenfels HM. Pulsed dye laser treatment is effective in the treatment of recalcitrant viral warts. Dermatologic Surgery. 2008;**34**(1):67-72

[82] Tan OT, Hurwitz RM, Stafford TJ. Pulsed dye laser treatment of recalcitrant verrucae: A preliminary report. Lasers in Surgery and Medicine. 1993;**13**(1):127-137

[83] Kenton-Smith J, Tan ST. Pulsed dye laser therapy for viral warts. British Journal of Plastic Surgery. 1999;**52**(7):554-558

[84] Vargas H, Hove CR, Dupree ML, Williams EF. The treatment of facial verrucae with the pulsed dye laser. Laryngoscope. 2002;**112**(9):1573-1576

[85] Grillo E, Boixeda P, Ballester A, Miguel-Morrondo A, Truchuelo T, Jaén P. Pulsed dye laser treatment for facial flat warts. Dermatologic Therapy. 2014;**27**(1):31-35

[86] van Brederode RL, Engel ED. Combined cryotherapy/70% salicylic acid treatment for plantar verrucae. The Journal of Foot and Ankle Surgery. 2001;**40**:36-41

[87] Wu C, Langan S, Kilmurray M, Lawlor D, Watson R. Efficacy of pulsed-dye laser for viral warts—An internal audit. Irish Medical Journal. 2003;**96**(80):82-83

[88] Kopera D. Verrucae vulgares: Flashlamp-pumped pulsed dye laser treatment in 134 patients. International Journal of Dermatology. 2003;**42**:905-908

[89] Tuncel A, Gorgu M, Ayhan M, Deren O, Erdogan B. Treatment of anogenital warts by pulsed dye laser. Dermatologic Surgery. 2002;**28**:350-352

[90] Khandpur S, SharmaVK. Efficacy of pulsed dye laser in cosmetically distressing facial dermatoses in skin types. Indian Journal of Dermatology. 2008;**53**(4):186-189

[91] Passeron T, Sebban K, Mantoux F, Fontas E, Lacour JP, Ortonne JP. Traitement des verrues palmo-plantaires par le laser à colorant pulsé à 595 nm: étude randomisée en simple insu contre placebo. Annales de Dermatologie et de Vénéréologie. 2007;**134**(2):135-139

[92] Akhyani M, Ehsani AH, Noormohammadpour P, Shamsodini R, Azizahari S, Sayanjali S. Comparing pulsed-dye laser with cryotherapy in the treatment of common warts. Journal of Lasers in Medical Sciences. 2010;**1**(1):14-19

[93] Akarsu S, Ilknur T, Demirtaşoglu M, Özkan S. Verruca vulgaris: Pulsed dye laser therapy compared with salicylic acid + pulsed dye laser therapy. Journal of the European Academy of Dermatology and Venereology. 2006;**20**(8):936-940

[94] Park HS, Choi WS. Pulsed dye laser treatment for viral warts: A study of 120 patients. The Journal of Dermatology. 2008;**35**(8):491-498

[95] Ross BS, Levine VJ, Nehal K, Tse Y, Ashinoff R. Pulsed dye laser treatment of warts: An update. Dermatologic Surgery. 1999;**25**(5):377-380

[96] Jain A, Storwick GS. Effectiveness of the 585 nm flashlamp-pulsed tunable dye laser (PTDL) for treatment of plantar verrucae. Lasers in Surgery and Medicine. 1997;**21**(5):500-505

[97] Sparreboom EF, Luiijks HG, Luiting-Welkenhuyzen HA, Willems PW, Groeneveld CP, Bovenschen HJ. Pulsed-dye laser

treatment for recalcitrant viral warts: A retrospective case seriesof 227 patients. The British Journal of Dermatology. 2014;**171**(5):1270-1273

[98] Pollock B, Sheehan-Dare R. Pulsed dye laser and intralesional bleomycin for treatment of resistant viol hand warts. Lasers in Surgery and Medicine. 2002;**30**(2):135-140

[99] Sethuraman G, Richards KA, Hiremagalore RN, Wagner A. Effectiveness of pulsed dye laser in the treatment of recalcitrant warts in children. Dermatologic Surgery. 2010;**36**(1):58-65

[100] Park HS, Kim JW, Jang SJ, Choi JC. Pulsed dye laser therapy for pediatric warts. Pediatric Dermatology. 2007;**24**(2):177-181

[101] Jacobsen E, McGraw R, McCagh S. Pulsed dye laser efficacy as initial therapy for warts and against recalcitrant verrucae. Cutis. 1997;**59**(4):206-208

[102] Kopera D. Verrucae vulgares: Flashlamp-pumped pulsed dye laser treatment in 134 patients. International Journal of Dermatology. 2003;**42**(11):905-908

[103] Dobson JS, Harland CC. Pulsed dye laser and intralesional bleomycin for the treatment of recalcitrant cutaneous warts. Lasers in Surgery and Medicine. 2014;**46**(2):112-116

[104] Gooptu C, James MP. Recalcitrant viral warts: Results of treatment with the KTP laser. Clinical and Experimental Dermatology. 1999;**24**:60-63

[105] Steele K, Irwin WG. Treatment options for cutaneous warts in family practice. Family Practice. 1988;**5**:314-319

[106] London ID. Buffered glutaraldehyde solution for warts. Archives of Dermatology. 1971;**104**:96-97

[107] Hirose R, Hori M, Shukuwa T, Udono M, Yamada M, Koide T, et al. Topical treatment of resistant warts with glutaraldehyde. The Journal of Dermatology. 1994;**21**:248-253

[108] Stonehill AA, Krop S, Borick PM. Buffered glutaraldehyde—A new chemical sterilizing solution. American Journal of Hospital Pharmacy. 1963;**20**:458-465

[109] Arýcan Ö. Verrukalarda güncel tedavi. Dermatose. 2004;**3**:159-159

[110] Mapar MA, Maghsoodi M, Maghsoodi K, Kardooni A, Shafiee A. Comparison between efficacy of formalin 5% solution and placebo in treatment of plane warts. Biomedical & Pharmacology Journal. 2017;**10**(1):81-87

[111] Sutana R, Alam M, Khondker L, Ahmed RS. Safety in use of cryotherapy and topical salicylic acid with lactic acid combination in treating verruca vulgaris. Mymensingh Medical Journal. 2012;**21**(4):715-722

[112] Bagwell A, Loy A, McFarland MS, Tessmer-Neubauer A. Oral acyclovir in the treatment of verruca. Journal of Drugs in Dermatology. 2016;**15**(2):237-238

[113] Tandeter H, Tandeter ER. Treatment of plantar warts with oral valacyclovir. The American Journal of Medicine. 01 June 2005;**118**(6):689-690. DOI: 10.1016/j.amjmed.2004.12.029. PMID: 15922706

[114] Hivnor C, Shepard JW, Shapiro MS, Vittorio CC, et al. Intravenous cidofovir for recalcitrant verruca vulgaris in the setting of HIV. Archives of Dermatology. 2004;**140**(1):13-14. DOI: 10.1001/archderm.140.1.13

[115] Turnbull JR, Husak R, Treudler R, Zouboulis CC, Orfanos CE. Regression of multiple viral warts in a human immunodeficiency virus-infected

patient treated by triple antiretroviral therapy. The British Journal of Dermatology. 2002;**146**:330

[116] Shumer SM, O'Keefe EJ. Bleomycin in the treatment of recalcitrant warts. Journal of the American Academy of Dermatology. 1983;**9**:91-96. [PubMed] [Google Scholar]

[117] van der Velden EM, Ijsselmuiden OE, Drost BH, Baruchin AM. Dermatography with bleomycin as a new treatment for verrucae vulgaris. International Journal of Dermatology. 1997;**36**:145-150

[118] Stulberg DL, Hutchinson AG. Molluscum contagiosum and warts. American Family Physician. 2003;**67**:1233-1240

[119] Stulberg DL, Hutchinson AG. Physicians need more evidence on treatments of warts: in reply. American Family Physician. 2003;**68**:1714-1716. Available from: http://www.aafp.org/afp/20031101/letters.html [Accessed: 10 May 2006]

[120] Sobh MA, Abd El-Razic MM, Rizc RA, Eid MM, Abd El-Hamid IA, Ghoneim MA. Intralesional injection of bleomycin sulphate into resistant warts in renal transplant recipients versus non-transplant warty patients. Acta Dermato-Venereologica. 1991;**71**:63-66

[121] James MP, Collier PM, Aherne W, Hardcastle A, Lovegrove S. Histologic, pharmacologic, and immunocytochemical effects of injection of bleomycin into viral warts. Journal of the American Academy of Dermatology. 1993;**28**:933-937

[122] Miller RA. Nail dystrophy following intralesional injections of bleomycin for aperiungual wart. Archives of Dermatology. 1984;**120**:963-964

[123] Yamamoto T. Bleomycin and the skin. The British Journal of Dermatology. 2006;**155**:869-875

[124] Abess A, Keel DM, Graham BS. Flagellate hyperpigmentation following intral-lesional bleomycin treatment of verruca plantaris. Archives of Dermatology. 2003;**139**:337-339

[125] Munn SE, Higgins E, Marshall M, et al. A new method of intralesional bleomycin therapy in the treatment of recalcitrant warts. The British Journal of Dermatology. 1996;**135**:969-971

[126] Loo S K-f, Tang W Y-m. Warts (non-genital). BMJ Clinical Evidence. 2014;**2014**:1710. PMCID: PMC4054795. PMID: 24921240

[127] Dhar SB, Rashid MM, Islam A, Bhuiyan M. Intralesional bleomycin in the treatment of cutaneous warts: A randomized clinical trial comparing it with cryotherapy. Indian Journal of Dermatology, Venereology and Leprology. 2009;**75**:262-267

[128] Seif R. Factors which disorganize microtubules or microfilaments increase the frequency of cell transformation by polyoma virus. Journal of Virology. 1980;**36**:421-428

[129] Krogh G. Penile condylomata acuminata an experimental model for evaluation of topical self-treatment with 0.5%-1.0% ethanolic preparations of podophyllotoxin for three days. Sexually Transmitted Diseases. 1981;**8**:179-186

[130] Gabriel G, Thin RNT. Treatment of anogerital warts: Comparison of trichloroacetic acid and podophyllin vs podophyllin alone. The British Journal of Venereal Diseases. 1983;**59**:124-126

[131] Workowski KA, Bolan GA. Sexually transmitted diseases treatment guidelines. Morbidity and mortality weekly report (MMWR). Recommendations and Reports. 5 June 2015;**64**(RR3):1-137. Available from: https://www.cdc.gov/mmwr/

[132] Briggs GC, Freeman RK, Yaffe SJ. Drugs in Pregnancy and Lactation.

9th ed. Philadelphia, PA: Lippincott Williams & Wilkins; 2011

[133] Hellberg D, Svarrer T, Nilsson S, Valentin J. Self-treatment of female external genital warts with 0.5% podophyllotoxin cream (Condyline) vs weekly applications of 20% podophyllin solution. International Journal of STD & AIDS. 1995;**6**:257-261

[134] Thappa DM, Chiramel MJ. Evolving role of immunotherapy in the treatment of refractory warts. Indian Dermatology Online Journal. 2016;**7**(5):364-370. DOI: 10.4103/2229-5178.190487

[135] Arndt KA, Bowers KE, Alam M, Reynolds R, Tsao S, editors. Warts. In: Manual of Dermatologic Therapeutics. 6th ed. Philadelphia: Lippincott Williams & Wilkins; 2002. pp. 241-251

[136] Moore RA, Edwards JE, Hopwood J, Hicks D. Imiquimod for the treatment of genital warts: Aquantitative systematic review. BMC Infectious Diseases. 2001;**1**:3. [PMC free article] [PubMed] [Google Scholar]

[137] Ahn CS, Huang WW. Imiquimod in the treatment of cutaneous warts: An evidence-based review. American Journal of Clinical Dermatology. 2014;**15**:387-399. [PubMed] [Google Scholar]

[138] Stefanaki C, Lagogiani I, Kouris A, Kontochristopoulos G, Antoniou C, Katsarou AJ. Cryotherapy versus imiquimod 5% cream combined with a keratolytic lotion in cutaneous warts in children: A randomized study. Journal of Dermatological Treatment. 2016;**27**(1):80-82. [PubMed] [Ref list]

[139] Ciavattini A, Tsiroglou D, Vichi M, Di Giuseppe J, Cecchi S, Tranquilli AL. Topical Imiquimod 5% cream therapy for external anogenital warts in pregnant women: Report of four cases and review of the literature. Journal of Maternal-Fetal and Neonatal Medicine. 2012;**25**(7):873-876. [PubMed] [Ref list]

[140] Garg S, Baveja S. Intralesional immunotherapy for difficult to treat warts with *Mycobacterium w* vaccine. Journal of Cutaneous and Aesthetic Surgery. 2014;**7**:203-208

[141] Singh S, Chouhan K, Gupta S. Intralesional immunotherapy with killed *Mycobacterium indicus pranii* vaccine for the treatment of extensive cutaneous warts. Indian Journal of Dermatology, Venereology and Leprology. 2014;**80**:509-514

[142] Gupta S, Malhotra AK, Verma KK, Sharma VK. Intralesional immunotherapy with killed *Mycobacterium w* vaccine for the treatment of ano-genital warts: An open label pilot study. Journal of the European Academy of Dermatology and Venereology: JEADV. 2008;**22**:1089-1093

[143] Meena JK, Malhotra AK, Mathur DK, Mathur DC. Intralesional immunotherapy with *Mycobacterium w* vaccine in patients with multiple cutaneous warts: Uncontrolled open study. JAMA Dermatology. 2013;**149**:237-239

[144] Dhakar AK, Dogra S, Vinay K, Sarangal R, Kanwar AJ, Singh MP. Intralesional *Mycobacterium w* vaccine versus cryotherapy in treatment of refractory extragenital warts: Arandomized, open-label, comparative study. Journal of Cutaneous Medicine and Surgery. 2016;**20**:123-129

[145] Kumar P, Dar L, Saldiwal S, Varma S, Datt Upadhyay A, Talwar D, et al. Intralesional injection of *Mycobacterium w* vaccine vs imiquimod, 5%, cream in patients with anogenital warts: Arandomized clinical trial. JAMA Dermatology. 2014;**150**:1072-1078

[146] Singh S, Chouhan K, Gupta S. Intralesional immunotherapy with

killed Mycobacterium indicus pranii vaccine for the treatment of extensive cutaneous warts. Indian Journal of Dermatology, Venereology and Leprology. 2014;**80**:509-514

[147] Zuo C, Huang J, Liao Z, Lu J, Chen J. Effects of BCG-PSN on serum levels of IL-4 and IL-12 in patients with condyloma acuminatum. Zhong Nan Da Xue Xue Bao. Yi Xue Ban. 2004;**29**:690-692

[148] Sharquie KE, Al-Rawi JR, Al-Nuaimy AA, Radhy SH. Bacille Calmette-Guerin immunotherapy of viral warts. Saudi Medical Journal. 2008;**29**:589-593

[149] Salem A, Nofal A, Hosny D. Treatment of common and plane warts in children with topical viable Bacillus Calmette-Guerin. Pediatric Dermatology. 2013;**30**:60-63

[150] Daulatabad D, Pandhi D, Singal A. BCG vaccine for immunotherapy in warts: Is it really safe in a tuberculosis endemic area? Dermatologic Therapy. 2016;**29**:168-172

[151] Zamanian A, Mobasher P, Jazi GA. Efficacy of intralesional injection of mumps-measles-rubella vaccine in patients with wart. Advanced Biomedical Research. 2014;**3**:107

[152] Nofal A, Nofal E. Intralesional immunotherapy of common warts: Successful treatment with mumps, measles and rubella vaccine. Journal of the European Academy of Dermatology and Venereology. 2010;**24**(10):1166-1170. DOI: 10.1111/j.1468-3083.2010.03611.x

[153] Kus S, Ergun T, Gun D, Akin O. Intralesional tuberculin for treatment of refractory warts. Journal of the European Academy of Dermatology and Venereology. 2005;**19**:515-516

[154] Clifton MM, Johnson SM, Roberson PK, et al. Immunotherapy for recalcitrant warts in children using intralesional mumps or Candida antigens. Pediatric Dermatology. 2003;**20**:268-271

[155] King M, Johnson SM, Horn TD. Intralesional immunotherapy for genital warts. Archives of Dermatology. 2005;**141**:1606-1607

[156] Signore RJ. Candida albicans intralesional injection immunotherapy of warts. Cutis. 2002;**70**:185-192

[157] Horn TD, Johnson SM, Helm RM, Roberson PK. Intralesional immunotherapy of warts with mumps, Candida and trichophyton skin test antigens: A single-blinded, randomized and controlled trial. Archives of Dermatology. 2005;**141**:589-594

[158] Johnson SM, Horn TD. Intralesional immunotherapy for warts using a combination of skin test antigens: A safe and effective therapy. Journal of Drugs in Dermatology. 2004;**3**:263-265

[159] Phillips RC, Ruhl TS, Pfenniger JL, Garber MR. Treatment of warts with Candida antigen injection. Archives of Dermatology. 2000;**136**:1274-1275

[160] Johnson SM, Roberson PK, Horn TD. Intralesional injection of mumps or Candida skin test antigens: A novel immunotherapy for warts. Archives of Dermatology. 2001;**137**:451-455

[161] Brunk D. Injection of Candida antigen works on warts. Skin Allergy News. 1999;**30**:5

[162] Majid I, Imran S. Immunotherapy with intralesional *Candida Albicans* antigen in resistant or recurrent warts: A study. Indian Journal of Dermatology. 2013;**58**(5):360-365

[163] Maronn M, Salm C, Lyon V, Galbraith S. One-year experience with Candida antigen immunotherapy

for warts and molluscum. Pediatric Dermatology. 2008;**25**:189-192

[164] Dianzani F. Viral interference and interferon. La Ricerca in Clinica e in Laboratorio. 1975;**5**:196-213. [PubMed] [Google Scholar]

[165] Turek LP, Byrne JC, Lowy DR, Dvoretzky I, Friedman RM, Howley PM. Interferon induces morphologic reversion with elimination of extrachromosomal viral genomes in bovine papillomavirus-transformed mouse cells. Proceedings of the National Academy of Sciences of the United States of America. 1982;**79**:7914-7918. DOI: 10.1073/pnas.79.24.7914. [PMC free article] [PubMed] [CrossRef] [Google Scholar]

[166] Yang J, Yu-guo P, Zeng Z-m, Yu Z-j, Huang N, Deng Q-w. Interferon for the treatment of genital warts: A systematic review. BMC Infectious Diseases. 2009;**9**:156

[167] Ibs KH, Rink L. Zinc-altered immune function. The Journal of Nutrition. 2003;**133**:1452S-1526S

[168] Fraker PJ, King LE. Reprogramming of the immune system during zinc deficiency. Annual Review of Nutrition. 2004;**24**:277-298

[169] Sharquie KE, Khorsheed AA, Al-Nuaimy AA. Topical zinc sulphate solution for treatment of viral warts. Saudi Medical Journal. 2007;**28**(9):1418-1421. View at Google Scholar; View at Scopus

[170] Khattar JA, Musharrafieh UM, Tamim H, Hamadeh GN. Topical zinc oxide vs salicylic acid-lactic acid combination in the treatment of warts. International Journal of Dermatology. 2007;**46**(4):427-430. View at Publisher; View at Google Scholar

[171] Al-Gurairi FT, Al-Waiz M, Sharquie KE. Oral zinc sulphate in the treatment of recalcitrant viral warts: Randomized placebo-controlled clinical trial. British Journal of Dermatology. 2002;**146**(3):423-431. View at Google Scholar

[172] Mun JH, Kim SH, Jung DS, et al. Oral zinc sulfate treatment for viral warts: An open-label study. Journal of Dermatology. 2011;**38**:541-545. View at Google Scholar

[173] Sharquine KA, Al-Nuaimy AA. Treatment of viral warts by intralesional injection of zinc sulphate. Annals of Saudi Medicine. 2002;**22**(1-2):26-28. View at Google Scholar; View at Scopus

[174] Paller AS. Cimetidine for the treatment of warts. The Western Journal of Medicine. 1996;**164**:520-521. [PMC free article] [PubMed] [Google Scholar]

[175] Mitsuishi T, Iida K, Kawana S. Cimetidine treatment for viral warts enhances IL-2 and IFN-gamma expression but not IL-18 expression in lesional skin. European Journal of Dermatology. 2003;**13**:445-448. [PubMed] [Google Scholar]

[176] Gooptu C, Higgins CR, James MP. Treatment of viral warts with cimetidine: An open-label study. Clinical and Experimental Dermatology. 2000;**25**:183-185. [PubMed] [Google Scholar]

[177] Yilmaz E, Alpsoy E, Basaran E. Cimetidine therapy for warts: Aplacebo-controlled, double-blind study. Journal of the American Academy of Dermatology. 1996;**34**:1005-1007. [PubMed] [Google Scholar]

[178] Rogers CJ, Gibney MD, Siegfried EC, Harrison BR, Glaser DA. Cimetidine therapy for recalcitrant warts in adults: Is it any better than placebo? Journal of the American Academy of Dermatology. 1999;**41**:123-127

[179] Karabulut AA, Sahin S, Eksioglu M. Is cimetidine effective for nongenital warts: A double-blind, placebo-controlled study. Archives of Dermatology. 1997;**133**:533-534

[180] Amer M, Tosson Z, Soliman A, Selim AG, Salem A, Al-Gendy AA. Verrucae treated by levamisole. International Journal of Dermatology. 1991;**30**:738-740. [PubMed] [Google Scholar]

[181] Moncada B, Rodriguez ML. Levamisole therapy for multiple warts. The British Journal of Dermatology. 1979;**101**:327-330. [PubMed] [Google Scholar]

[182] Saúl A, Sanz R, Gomez M. Treatment of multiple viral warts with levamisole. International Journal of Dermatology. 1980;**19**:342-343. [PubMed] [Google Scholar]

[183] Parsad D, Pandhi R, Juneja A, Negi KS. Cimetidine and levamisole versus cimetidine alone for recalcitrant warts in children. Pediatric Dermatology. 2001;**18**:349-352. [PubMed] [Google Scholar]

[184] Scheinfeld N, Rosenberg JD, Weinberg JM. Levamisole in dermatology: A review. American Journal of Clinical Dermatology. 2004;**5**:97-104. [PubMed] [Google Scholar]

[185] Markowitz LE, Tsu V, Deeks SL, et al. Human papillomavirus vaccine introduction—The first five years. Vaccine. 2012;**30**(Suppl 5):F139-F148

[186] Giuliano AR, Tortolero-Luna G, Ferrer E, et al. Epidemiology of human papillomavirus infection in men, cancers other than cervical and benign conditions. Vaccine. 2008;**26**(Suppl 10):K17-K28

[187] Blomberg M, Dehlendorff C, Sand C, Kjaer SK. Dose-related differences in effectiveness of human papillomavirus vaccination against genital warts: A nationwide study of 550,000 young girls. Clinical Infectious Diseases. 2015;**61**:676-682. [PubMed] [Google Scholar]

[188] Blomberg M, Dehlendorff C, Sand C, Kjaer SK. Dose-related differences in effectiveness of human papillomavirus vaccination against genital warts: A nationwide study of 550,000 young girls. Clinical Infectious Diseases. 2015;**61**:676-682. [PubMed] [Google Scholar]

[189] Chow EP, Read TR, Wigan R, Donovan B, Chen MY, Bradshaw CS, et al. Ongoing decline in genital warts among young heterosexuals 7 years after the Australian human papillomavirus (HPV) vaccination programme. Sexually Transmitted Infections. 2015;**91**:214-219. [PubMed] [Google Scholar]

[190] Shivakumar V, Okade R, Rajkumar V. Autoimplantation therapy for multiple warts. Indian Journal of Dermatology, Venereology and Leprology. 2009;7:593-595

[191] Das S, Das S, Chowdhury J, Patra S, Ghoshal L, Banerjee S. Auto-wart inoculation: An easy and effective treatment of multiple, recalcitrant and genital warts. Journal of Pakistan Association of Dermatologists. 2016;**26**(3):229-234

[192] Buckley DA, Keane FM, Munn SE, Fuller LC, Higgins EM, Du Vivier AW. Recalcitrant viral warts treated by diphencyprone immunotherapy. The British Journal of Dermatology. 1999;**141**:292-296

[193] Upitis JA, Krol A. The use of diphenylcyclopropenone in the treatment of recalcitrant warts. Journal of Cutaneous Medicine and Surgery. 2002;**6**:214-217

[194] Focht DR 3rd, Spicer C, Fairchok MP. The efficacy of duct tape vs cryotherapy in the treatment of verruca vulgaris (the common wart). Archives of Pediatrics & Adolescent Medicine. 2002;**156**:971-974

[195] Seki T, Tsuji K, Hayato Y, Moritomo T, Ariga T. Garlic and onion oils inhibit proliferation and induce differentiation of HL-60 cells. Cancer Letters. 2000;**160**:29-35

[196] Zedan H, Hofny ERM, Ismail SA. Propolis as an alternative treatment for cutaneous warts. International Journal of Dermatology. 2009;**48**:1246-1249. [PubMed] [Google Scholar]

[197] Gupta AK, Daigle D. Sinecatechins 10% ointment: A green tea extract for the treatment of external genital warts. Skin Therapy Letter. 2015;**20**:6-8. [PubMed] [Google Scholar]

[198] Domínguez Gómez J, Simón RD, Abreu Daniel A, Zelenkova H. Effectiveness of glycyrrhizinic Acid (glizigen) and an immunostimulant (viusid) to treat anogenital warts. ISRN Dermatology. 2012;**2012**:863692. DOI: 10.5402/2012/863692

[199] Kolev N, Bakardzhiev I. Glycyrrhizinic acid—An alternative treatment of anogenital warts during pregnancy. European Journal of Obstetrics, Gynecology, and Reproductive Biology. 2016;**206**:e86

[200] Kavya M, Shashikumar BM, et al. Safety and efficacy of intralesional vitamin D3 in cutaneous warts: An open uncontrolled trial. Journal of Cutaneous and Aesthetic Surgery. 2017;**10**(2):90-94

Chapter 4

Human Papillomavirus Infections in Pregnant Women and Its Impact on Pregnancy Outcomes: Possible Mechanism of Self-Clearance

Sanchita Roy Pradhan, Sutapa Mahata, Dipanwita Ghosh, Pranab Kumar Sahoo, Sinjini Sarkar, Ranita Pal and Vilas D. Nasare

Abstract

Young women are at the maximum risk of Human papillomavirus (HPV) infection which are asymptomatic in a majority of cases and spontaneously get cleared. Women in the age between 20 and 35 years are more active sexually and especially in the developing nations, this age group forms a major cohort among the population of pregnant women. The changed hormonal *milieu* and immune response during pregnancy might favor presence or persistence of HPV infection, while at the same time natural clearance also takes place during pregnancy with an unknown mechanism. Various HPVs have been reported to be associated with preterm rupture of membranes (PROM), fetal growth restriction (FGR), preeclampsia, placental abnormalities and preterm delivery in several populations. The risk factors involved in the intrauterine environment affects fetal development and thus increase the development risk of specific diseases in adult life as per the hypothesis of the fetal origins of adult disease (FOAD). The structural and molecular changes in the feto-maternal interface support and protect the semiallogeneic fetus from immune-mediated or inflammatory injury. On the other hand, the trophoblast cells of placenta facilitate the replication of HPV and the affliction of placenta and the vaginal infection can directly be associated with pregnancy outcomes. So, to optimize better child health care and reproductive outcomes, HPV screening might help during pregnancy. It is therefore important to understand how the HPV is affecting the early pregnancy and immune cells within the feto-maternal interface are educated for self-clearance to fulfill their biological functions or prevalence to affect the pregnancy outcomes and how the persistence of HR-HPV infection overtime increases the development of cervical cancer risk.

Keywords: pregnancy, self clearance, feto-maternal cell trafficking, HPV vaccine, cervical cancer

1. Introduction

The most common sexually transmitted infectious conditions across the globe are Human papillomavirus (HPV) infections which is responsible for the development of cervical cancer. The infection of HPV does not always lead towards the neoplastic disease which suggests that the clearance or acquisition of HPV infections may depend on the interpersonal variations in the immune system as well as environmental or viral factors. For example, a well-established cervical cancer risk factor is parity. However, the influence of pregnancy in the natural history of HPV infection and thus the development of cervical neoplasia and its exact mechanism is not known [1].

At the beginning of the pregnancy, immune modulation and induction of tolerance are required for successful implantation allowance but as the pregnancy progresses a responsive immune system is responsible for a successful pregnancy which can protect both the fetus and the mother against environmental insults whenever there is a necessity arises. Indeed the maternal immune system reinforces networks that can respond according to the recognized danger signals and eliminate them appropriately promoting repair when needed. Not only the maternal immune system but also the actively developing immune system in the fetal-placental unit can modify further the maternal immune response and the reaction of the maternal immune system to the environment. So, the immunity during pregnancy is dynamic and unique which can be modulated as per the requirement and definitely not suppressed [2].

Several studies have proven the idea incorrect that constant immunosuppression is crucial for a successful pregnancy which demonstrates that inhibition of key signaling pathways such as pathways mediated by FAS; FAS ligand and deletion of immune cells at the implantation site are detrimental to pregnancy which may lead to pregnancy loss [3, 4]. The deletion of specific decidual NK cells leads to poor endometrial vascularity and obstruct the invasion of the trophoblast [5]. Thus, for a successful pregnancy the presence of immune infiltrates is required which suggests that the immune cells are not recruited to the decidua as a response to a 'non-self' or 'foreign' fetus but recruited actively to facilitate proper implantation and promote successful pregnancy.

During pregnancy and postpartum, different levels of hormonal changes and changes in the immunity may be responsible for the modulation of the natural history of the HPV infection. There are differences in the status of HPV infection during pregnancy and reduction in the number of HPV positive cases during postpartum period have been reported by various authors [6]. Though the dynamics of HPV infection during pregnancy is not well understood and the information remains controversial. The clearance and persistence of HPV during and after pregnancy have been studied by very few authors [7].

HPV infection in most cases naturally disappears in a short relative time period and risk of disease development in that case is very less. As pregnancy affects the host immune system, it is believed that pregnancy reduces the seroreactivity against infection of HPV. The upstream regulatory region of HPV18 has been reported to be activated by estrogen and progesterone which alters the clearance rate of HPV compared to non-pregnant women [8]. HPV genotypes and viral characteristics such as population distribution and evasive ability play an important role during persistent infection. However, how the HPV genotype specific reaction of the host immune system and the sexual behavior of pregnant women affect the rates of infection in case of persistent cases and how it is related to the host in not clear [9].

In pregnancy, the pregnant mother which is an adult organism is exposed to the fetus which is partly an extremely young organism and this phenomenon can be viewed similar to a natural state known as parabiosis in which organisms share partly blood systems. However, the fetus may have restoring effect on the maternal system. It has been reported that the regenerative capacity of the aged liver and other organs in mice model is restored by pregnancy [10].

There are controversial results on the risk of HPV infection in pregnant women. A higher HPV prevalence has been reported in few studies in pregnant women, whereas, some claimed there are no statistical difference among the age matched non-pregnant women [9]. Moreover, there are no studies on estimating the trimester, age and type specific prevalence of cervical HPV DNA in pregnant women.

This chapter will focus on the incidence of HPV infection in pregnant women population, the reason behind higher incidence rates in early pregnancy, the possible mechanisms responsible for self-clearance and non-clearance of HPV in pregnant women, immune mechanisms playing role in pregnancy, feto-maternal cell trafficking and how HPV affects the pregnancy outcomes. Furthermore, we will also discuss the potential of HPV infection during pregnancy can lead to the development of cervical cancer and therapeutic strategies.

2. Incidence of HPV infection in pregnant women population

Highest incidence rates have been reported in young adults just after the onset of their sexual activity [11]. In young women between the age group of 17 and 24 years, longitudinal studies reported incidence rates of HPV infection ranging from 15.7 to 29.4 of all types per 1000 women-months [12]. Women in their thirties showed a lower incidence rate in cohort studies which is between 5.2 and 13.4 any type HPV infection per 1000 women-months [12]. The prevalence is likewise higher in younger age groups than older. The global HPV prevalence estimated by a multi-country meta-analysis is 11.7% (with confidence interval 95% 11.6–11.7%) with normal cytology in women with an important variation within and between geographic regions. At round 25 years the prevalence peaks and decreases thereafter. It has been reported that at around 45 years a smaller second peak is observed [13, 14]. It has also been reported in various studies that within 1–2 years of HPV infection almost 80% of them resolve spontaneously [15]. Various studies suggested that during pregnancy it is more likely to acquire and progress HPV infection [16] which regresses after delivery [6, 7, 17, 18].

Whereas, Liu et al. [16] reported that in pregnant women the HPV prevalence varies from 9.58 to 46.67% and in age-matched non-pregnant women the prevalence varies from 8.9 to 23.5%, with a summary estimate of 16.82 and 12.25% respectively and there are significant differences between the summary estimates. In Asia, North America and Europe, it has been reported that the HPV prevalence rates are significantly higher in pregnant women as compared to those in non-pregnant women and the pregnant women in North America as compared to those in Europe and Asia are more susceptible to HPV infection [16]. As per the meta-analytical data showed by Liu et al. [16], the prevalence rates of HPV infection in pregnant women in North America, Australia, Europe and Asia were 30.37, 36.60, 13.19 and 15.72% respectively which showed a worldwide significant difference. In pregnant women aged 25, 25–29 and $\geq$ 30 years the prevalence rates of HPV infection were 23.94, 13.34 and 14.79% respectively and in non-pregnant women the prevalence rates were 18, 12.08 and 11.43% in respective three age groups [16]. The most frequently identified HPV types in pregnant women have been reported are HPV-16 with 3.86% prevalence rate, HPV-6 with 2.45% prevalence rate, HPV-18 with 1.80% prevalence rate and HPV-11 with 1.76% prevalence rate which is as same as the prevalence rates in non-pregnant women of these HPV types. In the three trimesters the HPV prevalence rates reported are 18.20, 14.38 and 19.32% and the odd ratios are 1.59, 1.20 and 1.71 respectively as compared to the non-pregnant women population.

Studies conducted in Hong Kong and Hungary showed that in asymptomatic pregnant women HPV-16 is the most common type and HPV-6,-18,-11,-58,-31 and – 33 are the other common HPV types [19]. Whereas, in non-pregnant women the sequence is bit different such as HPV-16, -6, -11, -18, -58, -33 and -31 and in women with normal cytology worldwide the sequence reported is HPV-16, -18, -31, -58 and -52 [16].

Specific to genital tract infections, HPV types are classified into three risk categories based on their relative malignant potential such as HPV-6, -11, -40, -42, -43, -44 are low risk; HPV-31, -33, -35, -51, -52 are intermediate and HPV-16, -18, -45, -56 are high risk types. Young women between the ages of 10 and 35 years are reported to be at the maximum risk of HPV infection which are asymptomatic in majority of the cases and spontaneously get cleared may be due to the strong immune system. The reason being this is the age when women are sexually more active. A major cohort of the pregnant population is formed by this age group in the developing nations. The changed immune response and hormonal *milieu* during pregnancy might favor the presence or persistence of the HPV infection. Niyibizi et al. [18] reported the prevalence of HPV infection in pregnant women with a wide variation from 5.5 to 65%. Various HPVs in several populations have been reported to be associated with adverse pregnancy outcomes such as preeclamsia, preterm rupture of membranes (PROM), preterm delivery, fetal growth restriction and placental abnormalities. However, no such data on the association of the HPV infection in pregnancy and its outcome from the Indian subcontinent is available till date [20].

3. The reason behind higher incidence rates in early pregnancy

3.1 Maternal immunity during pregnancy

Starting at the conception and towards the course of completion with labor and birth enormous transformations the uterus has to undergo in pregnancy. In order to achieve blastocyst stage embryo development for a newly fertilized egg and successful invasion into the uterine tissue, there is a requirement of finely balanced subsets of immune cells and their soluble mediators. Mainly genetics determine the developmental potential of the blastocyst. However, the optimal environment of the uterus determines the viability and competence of the blastocyst to become a fully developed fetus and on-time delivery achievements which in turn reflects the maternal immune response quality.

It has been claimed that pregnancy is a state of mild immunosuppression due to the reduction in the helper T-cell type 1 cell mediated response or decrease in natural killer cells. Sillman and Sedlis in the year 1987 reported that a higher incidence of cervical neoplasia is found in immunosuppressed women [15]. A steroidal hormone receptor binding element present on the transcriptional promotor of HPV-16 as reported by Gloss et al. is responsible for promotion of HPV transcription which suggests an involvement of hormonal activation of replication of HPV [21]. Observation from various studies indicated that the temporary altered immunity state and the increased steroidal hormonal levels during pregnancy might have an influence of the subsequence progression of the disease development effecting on HPV replication [16].

Fetus inherits 50% genome from the father that leads to the expressing of antigens which are acknowledged as foreign by the maternal immune system. To accommodate the semi-allogeneic fetus within the immunocompetent mother's body a range of complex processes take place [22]. The physiological and immunological changes during pregnancy marks it a unique condition that makes the mother and the fetus more susceptible to certain infectious diseases, risk of congenital anomalies and the risk of more serious outcomes in other diseases. These changes are mainly driven by the cytokines, hormones and immune cells that lead to the modification of the immune system as well as the structural changes by remodeling of the endometrium [23]. In the 1950s, it was initially proposed that the induction of general immunosuppression during pregnancy allows the tolerance of the semi-allogeneic fetus and since then several hypotheses has been proposed explaining the reason why the fetus is not rejected by the maternal immune system (**Figure 1**).

On the contrary, after the natural infection pregnant women are capable of inducing immune responses and immune memory which is similar to non-pregnant women which proves the above hypothesis wrong [24]. Various studies have reported that the modulation of the immune system rather than active suppression is observed during pregnancy. Over the course of pregnancy, the progressive increase of the concentrations of steroidal hormones such as progesterone and estrogens induce a shift in the balance of pro and anti-inflammatory responses. During the first trimester of pregnancy which is called "open wound phase" the pro-inflammatory responses are prominent and in the second and the third trimester phases where the body prepared for deliver the anti-inflammatory responses are prominent [22]. Thus, it is clear that why the severity of certain diseases such as multiple sclerosis, rheumatoid arthritis induced by the inflammatory responses are often gets reduced during the third trimester of pregnancy and diseases which are controlled by the inflammatory responses such as malaria, influenza and lupus are increased during this phase [25]. There is a shift from Th1, which is oriented towards cell-mediated immunity, towards Th2, which is oriented towards the hormonal immunity, responses is observed which is associated with an alteration of the balance between type1 and type 2T helper cells and this transition is needed for the development of a healthy fetus. The suppression of cytotoxic T lymphocytes and stimulation of B lymphocytes to further increase the production of antibodies that are potential to be transferred to the fetus is controlled by these Th2-skewed responses. The findings of Mor et al. [22] and Chaouat et al. [24] suggested that the placenta is capable of interaction and response to pathogens which makes it an active immunological site. At the feto-maternal interphase, the immune mechanisms contribute to protect the fetus from rejection providing required cytokines and growth factors for implantation of the fetus in the

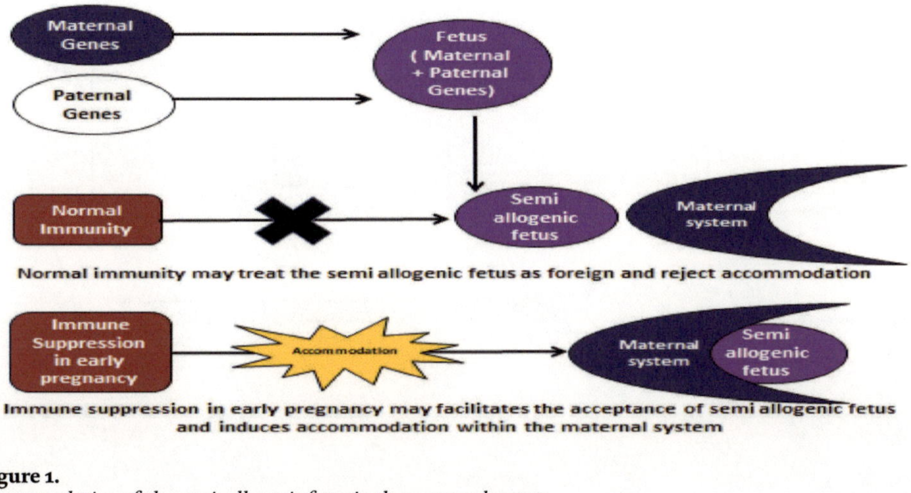

Figure 1.
Accommodation of the semi-allogenic fetus in the maternal system.

placenta. The placenta can generate signals which may modulate the responses of the maternal immune system to pathogens which leads to a new paradigm that there is a combination of signals and responses originating both from the feto-placental unit and the maternal immune system which decides the overall immunological responses during pregnancy (**Figure 2**) [26].

3.2 Anatomical changes during pregnancy

The increased susceptibility to infection of pregnant women during pregnancy may be due to the immunological and anatomical changes of the uterine canal. Like other human viruses, the placenta or the cells of the fetal origin may get infected by HPV. The presence of HPV has been reported in the polymorphonuclear cells which suggest that the passage of virus through feto-maternal barrier may be allowed by the transfer of the maternal cells [27]. It has also been reported that the trophoblast cells are broadly permissive *in vitro* for HPV and within the trophoblast cell cultures this virus is able to complete its life cycle [28, 29].

In the uterine mucosa, especially in the postovulatory phase there is an increase in the circulating progesterone levels which initiates a cascade of molecular and cellular events that allows the initial anchor of the embryo to the epithelial layer of the endometrial surface further leading to the coordination of the invasion of the extra-embryonic trophoblast lineages. The proliferative activity of estrogen-primed endometrium is inhibited by progesterone which induces the secretory activity in the glandular compartment followed by triggering the influx of specialized uterine natural killer cells such as uNK; CD16/CD56bright in response to the production of local chemokines such as CXCL9, CCL4 and CXCL10. The Uterine natural killer (uNK) cells which are a rich source of angiogenic and growth factors, has been reported to have critical role in remodeling of the endometrial spiral arteries during and prior to pregnancy [5, 30]. The contractile activity of the myocytes of the junctional zone is strongly reduced by the progesterone which is a crucial process for the apposition of the blastocyst to the luminal epithelium. The most outstanding aspect of the maternal response during pregnancy is the transformation of the endometrial stromal fibroblasts into epithelioid-like, secretory decidual cells.

Upon implantation of a blastocyst, decidualization of the stromal compartment is observed in most species. On the other hand, in humans decidualization is initiated without the involvement of a pregnancy in the midsecretory phase of the cycle. It is progressive process which is at first initiated around the terminal spiral arteries

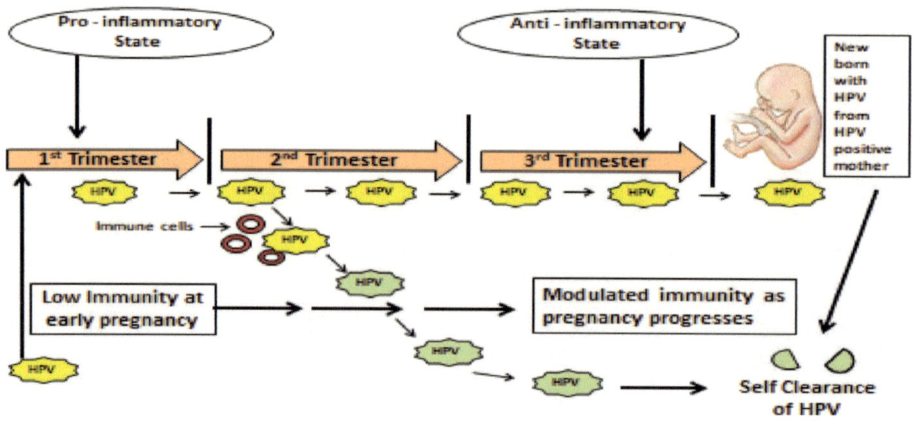

Figure 2.
HPV clearance and non-clearance during pregnancy and postpartum.

of the superficial endometrial layer which continues in pregnancy involving the entire endometrium as the pregnancy progresses [23]. The invasive or extravillous trophoblastic cells mediate the attachment of the placenta to the maternal uterine wall and they are responsible for the establishment of a low-resistance, high-flow supply of the maternal circulation to the fetus and the placenta. The placental dysfunction occurs due to the failed invasion of the extravillous trophoblast cells leading to the adverse obstetric outcomes such as spontaneous preterm delivery and pre-eclampsia. There are controversial reports on the HPV infection of the invasive trophoblast cells and their effects. There are reports showing the evidence of detection of HPV in trophoblast tissue from early pregnancy losses where HPV was more prominently found in spontaneous abortion cases than in cases of elective terminations of pregnancy. The genomes of the four different HPV types such as 11, 18, 16 and 31 are reported to undergo complete life cycle in 3A trophoblast cell lines and the HPV-31 in an in vitro system are shown to decrease cell number of the trophoblast cell and their adhesion [31].

Impaired placental function is associated with pregnancy loss or complications such as abruption, fetal growth restriction and pre-eclampsia. In this case we have to consider that the uterine remodeling during pregnancy is required to accommodate deep trophoblast invasion and the decidual process is not primary under the embryonic control which makes the implantation process more vulnerable to perturbations in the mother [23].

4. The possible mechanisms responsible for self-clearance and non-clearance of HPV in pregnant women

4.1 Role of maternal immunity

Between the maternal decidua and the blastocyst the first point of contact is represented by the trophoblast. It has been reported by current studies that the trophoblast plays an active role during implantation and early placentation in shaping the immunological milieu by educating and attracting immune cells at the implantation site and thus modeling the subsequent response of the immune cells to external stimuli. Cytokines such as transforming growth factor-β (TGF β), CXCL12 which is also known as SDF1, CXCL8 which is also known as IL-8 and CCL2 which is also known as MCP1 are constitutively secreted by trophoblast cells. The secretion of these cytokines by trophoblast cells upon establishment at the implantation site, promotes the recruitment of neutrophils, peripheral monocytes, T cells, NK cells and Treg cells [32]. After decidualization although immune infiltrates are already present, studies have shown that for successful pregnancy, immune cell trafficking is crucial and any disruption in these chemokines signaling pathways leads to reduced infiltration of the immune cells and adverse pregnancy outcomes. Cytokines are also secreted by trophoblast cells that can act on immune cells after their recruitment. These secreted cytokines have been reported to stimulate the unique differentiation of the earlier recruited immune cells in such as a way that they acquire phenotypes which are collectively essential for the successful pregnancy [33].

Decidual NK cells are less cytotoxic, thus they are different from peripheral NK cells and TGFβ12 and trophoblast-derived IL-15 induces this type of phenotypes. Decidual vascular remodeling which is crucial for development of the placenta targeted by these specialized NK cells [34]. CD14+ monocytes upon recruitment to the maternal-fetal interface acquire a unique phenotype that is M2-like macrophage which might be induced by the trophoblast-derived macrophage colony-stimulating factor (M-CSF) and IL-10 [2118]. These M2-like macrophages participate in clearance of apoptotic cells and phagocytosis of degraded extracellular matrix and play a crucial role in tissue remodeling [35]. Trophoblast-educated M2 like macrophages on the contrary to other tissue-resident macrophages, maintain their CD14 expression and capable of immunomodulatory cytokine secretions such as type I interferons and TGFβ [35]. Trophoblast-derived TGFβ furthermore is able to induce the naive CD4+ cell differentiation into FOXP3+ Treg cells [36]. In addition to the trophoblast cells, a substantial amount of data have shown that the decidual cells also have vital role in regulation of the immune cell trafficking which is mostly T cells towards the site of implantation (**Figure 3**) [37, 38].

In addition to chemokines and cytokines secretion which attract and educate immune cells, numerous studies have shown that the trophoblast cells have the ability to sense and respond according to the microenvironment. Cell-surface receptors expressed by the trophoblast cells such as NOD-like receptors (NLRs) and TLRs can recognize specific molecular patterns within the microenvironment. These receptors have also the ability to recognize DAMPs which are basically released from damaged tissues and dying cells as well as PAMPs (Pathogen-associated molecular patterns) from viruses, bacteria and other microorganisms and thus permit the trophoblast cells to sense and response to these signals [39, 40]. Thus, the placental and fetal development is supported by the trophoblast cells attracting and educating immune cells and responding to the signals within the microenvironment in a unique way such as decidual differentiation followed by trophoblast migration and invasion, angiogenesis and finally spiral artery remodeling [41].

4.2 How pregnancy responses to viral infections

During pregnancy the consequences of viral infection can vary being a benign asymptomatic event which is undetected mostly and it can either cause the occurrence of fetal congenital malformations or pregnancy loss [42]. Like bacteria, the TLRs and NLRs expressed by the immune cells as well as those expressed by the trophoblast cells can be engaged by the viruses. Viral replication as well as vertical transmission of a virus to the developing fetus from the mother can also controlled by the trophoblast cells [43, 44]. Commensal bacteria which are present at the

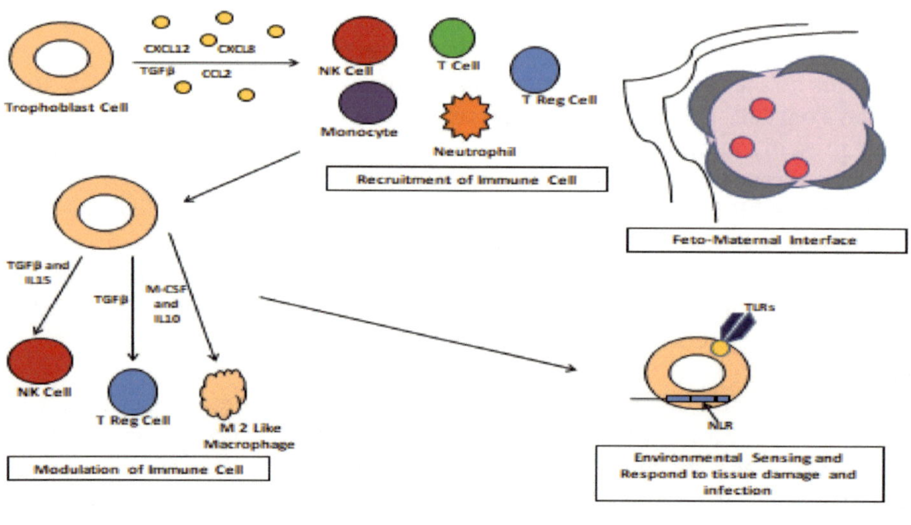

Figure 3.
Immune modulation during pregnancy at the feto-maternal interface.

feto-maternal interface can induce the secretion of IFNβ by trophoblast cells which supports the decidual receptivity by exerting immunomodulatory effects. It has been reported that the antiviral responses can be exerted by the IFNβ [45] and thus one of the molecular pathways that is type I IFN pathway is actively inhibited by the viruses as they establish as infection. Various studies in mouse model have demonstrated that by inhibiting IRF3 phosphorylating in the placenta, viral infection can decrease IFNβ expression which leads to the decreased antiviral responses [46]. TLR4 induced responses are modified by viral infections to commensal bacteria leading to the conversion of pro-inflammatory from anti-inflammatory in nature [47]. The receptivity and tolerance at the feto-maternal interface is promoted by the IFNβ which suggests that blunted response of IFNβ secondary to viral infection is responsible for the detrimental pregnancy consequences. The reduced receptivity of the immune cells at the feto-maternal interface due to the loss of IFNβ also reduces their capacity to control and respond to other microorganisms. Thus, the association of the overwhelming inflammation with pregnancy complications suggests that there may be an involvement of an undetected viral infection which can change the response pattern of the feto-maternal interface to commensal bacteria. This hypothesis has been supported by the study results of Cardenas et al. [48] using an animal model. In that study, pregnant C57BL/6 mice was infected with MHV68 on 8.5 embryonic day and a low dose of LPS subsequent administration on E15.5 day leads to a cytokine storm which was characterized by high levels of G-CSF, CXCL1, IL-8 and TNF which is associated with parturition, a reduced production of IFNβ followed by preterm birth. These changes in the cytokine profile leading to preterm birth is not induced alone either by LPS treatment or MHV68 infection but by a 'double-hit hypothesis' proposed by Mor et al. [41] which suggests that how trophoblast cells respond to bacterial products are changed by a viral infection which abolishes the normal microbiota immunomodulatory effects. In response of the commensal microbiota, the trophoblastic cells in the absence of a viral infection secret IFNβ, whereas IFNβ signaling is abolished in the presence of a viral infection leading to eradicate its immunomodulatory effects which in turn changes the response of the trophoblastic cells to commensal bacteria shifting IFNβ response to a cytokine storm which promotes preterm birth. However, it has been reported that the inflammation and preterm labour is also promoted either by an increased response of IFNβ or inhibition of the IFNβ regulators [49]. Thus, the original milieu which has a setting of immune-tolerance, during viral infection, is shifted into a state of pro-inflammatory condition [41].

4.3 Role of feto-maternal cell trafficking

During pregnancy there is a bidirectional cell passage exists between fetus and mother which is called feto-maternal cell trafficking. It is known as fetal microchimerism when there is a presence of fetal cells in the maternal circulation and maternal microchimerism when the maternal cells are present in the fetal circulation. Georg Schmorl in the year 1893 first reported about fetal microchimerism after identifying the placental trophoblast cells in a mother who died due to eclampsia [50]. The persistence of fetal cells in the maternal circulation [51, 52] and other maternal organs such as liver, heart, kidney [52] and bone marrow [53] has been reported decades after pregnancy. In 1963, with the identification of the maternal platelets and leukocytes in the cord blood the maternal microchimerism was described for the first time [54]. In healthy, immunocompetent individuals these maternal cells have been found to circulate into adult life [55].

At 7 weeks of pregnancy the bidirectional trafficking of the cells begins and increases throughout the gestation steadily and peaks at parturition [56]. In normal pregnancies, maternal microchimerism and fetal microchimerism has been reported to be 42 and 51% respectively at the time of delivery [57]. In human blood and tissues the detection of maternal-fetal microchimerism is done by in situ hybridization for identification of whole cells and the identification of the origin of the DNA whether it is from mother or the fetus is done by polymerase chain reaction (PCR) to identify Y-chromosome DNA sequences in mother [58]. As the Y chromosome is easier to distinguish it is used as a biomarker to detect microchimerism and it does not require the fetus to be male. However, male microchimerism has been reported to be found in a fifth of women with no birth of a male child. The possible reason of the phenomenon can be a vanished male twin; early miscarriage of a male embryo; transfer of male cell through the maternal circulation from an older sibling to a later pregnancy; or due to an unexplored possibility of transfer of male DNA into the maternal circulation during sexual intercourse [59]. In females, male fetal cells have reported to show increased antigenicity. As the fetus carries paternal genes among which some are expressed on the cell surface that may induce potent allogeneic responses the mother confronts an immunological challenge during pregnancy. However, in spite of the immunologic differences of the cells, the fetus does not get rejected frequently (**Figure 4**) [60].

In pregnancy, the maternal and fetal cell exchange is common. During gestation, placenta allows the fetal and maternal reciprocal transport of cells in a state of mutual tolerance which proves placenta is not an immunologically inert barrier. It is not necessary to continue a pregnancy and deliver a child to develop mirochimerism. Up to 500,000 nucleated fetal cells can be delivered into the maternal circulation even early terminations from surgical abortion [61, 62]. The cellular movement across the placental barrier is controlled by the maternal, fetal, or/and placental signals rather than nonspecific leakiness. The involvements of integrin-dependent and VEGF pathways are associated with the trans-placental cell trafficking mechanism but the initiation of the processes by the exact molecular signals are yet unknown [63]. In case of preeclampsia, fetal surgery and pregnancy termination where there is a disruption of the feto-maternal interface, association of altered feto-maternal cell trafficking has been reported which suggests that the placenta has a role in the cell migration regulation. The altered microchimerism levels are also associated with histocompatibility differences which suggests that the cell trafficking and the survival of the trafficked cells is either promoted or hindered by the immune response between the fetus and the mother [64, 65]. During pregnancy, the biological role of the bidirectional movement of cells is unknown, although it has implications in the fetal immune system development [66]; repair of tissue in autoimmune disease [67–70] tolerance mechanisms during pregnancy [71]; immune surveillance

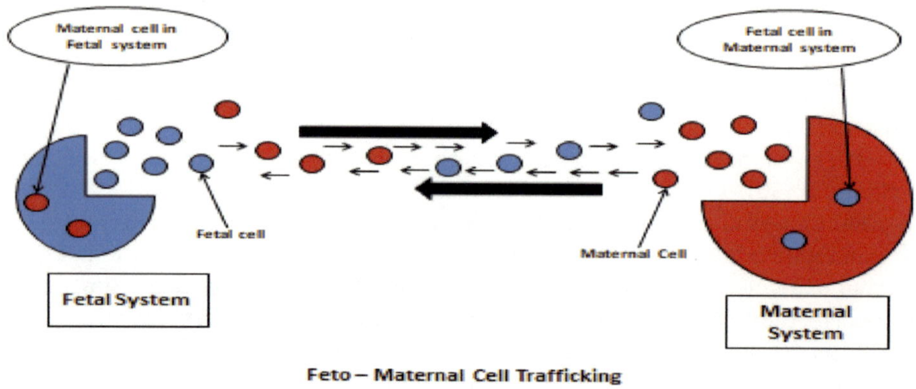

Figure 4.
Feto-maternal cell trafficking during pregnancy.

[72] and cancer [73]. It is also involved in the maintenance of balance between the tolerance [74] and immunologic priming [75] which can influence the occurrence of autoimmune disease and transplantation outcomes. The utility of the feto-maternal cell trafficking has been identified clinically in the prediction of pregnancy complications [76, 77] and in prenatal testing for aneuploidies [78].

The research on microchimerism is still in its infancy, more specifically on the fetomaternal microchimerism. In women with autoimmune diseases, the long-term existence of the fetal cells and its speculative role has not yet been studied well. It has been reported by some of the researchers that the microchimeric cell populations occur due to pregnancy may have stem cell like properties which have the potential to home in damaged tissues and organs and further differentiate as part of the maternal repair response [62].

5. How HPV affects the pregnancy outcomes

Merckx et al. [79] reported that children born to HPV-positive mothers are at a significantly higher risk of becoming HPV positive which further results in infantile genital and anal condyloma acuminatum and juvenile laryngeal papillomatosis. However, by the age of 6 months some HPV infections are almost cleared. Hence, the question regarding susceptibility of pregnant women to HPV infection and its prevalence as compared to non-pregnant women population are crucial to answer [16].

Various studies reported that spontaneous abortion occurs in up to 30% of all pregnancies and it constitutes one of the most frequently occurring adverse pregnancy outcomes worldwide. In 5–13% of deliveries, spontaneous preterm birth is also observed [80]. As per the reports of recent investigations, the human papillomavirus infection of the placenta may be involved with placental abnormalities, spontaneous preterm delivery and spontaneous abortion.

Trophoblast cells as discussed earlier constitute the prime target for HPV in placenta which is responsible for placentation abnormality. Various studies showed that in pregnant women the prevalence of HPV infection ranges widely from 6 to 65% and the HPV DNA has been detected in amniotic fluid, placenta, fetal membranes and umbilical cord blood [81].

Delivery before 37 weeks of gestation is defined as preterm birth and it is an important complication worldwide for both multifetal and singleton pregnancies. As compared to children born at term, the preterm children are more likely to develop log-term neurological and developmental disorders and are at an increased risk of mortality. The highest rates of preterm delivery have been reported to be found in South-eastern and South Asia with a percentage of 13.4%. Especially in low-income countries, the morbidity and mortality are highest among these preterm children [80].

As per the fetal origin of adult disease (FOAD) hypothesis, the specific changes in the fetus are caused by the intrauterine environmental exposures which lead to the risk of developing diseases in adult life. Depending on the environmental interaction, these risks may lead to adult diseases. Coronary heart disease was documented earlier to support this hypothesis [82] but a range of chronic conditions has also now been included to expand the framework [83]. While, the 'thrifty phenotype' hypothesis states that low birth weight babies should not be at high risk of non-insulin dependent diabetes development when they grow with a scarcity of food [84, 85] but growing up in an area of affluence of the same babies would increase the risk and hence the intrauterine exposure plays an important role in inheriting the harmful potential in interaction with exposures later. Thus, the reformulated FOAD hypothesis included epigenetics and the life –course epidemiology as an important factor which includes social and physical exposures during gestation, adolescence, childhood, young adulthood and adult life. To understand the development of chronic diseases, history specific and inter-generational elements of individual's life is also important [86]. The timing of exposure variables and how the outcome of interest is related to each other is the basis of life-course perspective. Hence, the effects of intrauterine exposures can be modified by the entire lifespan of an individual through the life-events, behavioral, biological and socioeconomic processes [87].

Infection with HPV (Human papillomavirus) is generally regarded as sexually transmitted disease. However, the detection of HPV in the oral mucosa of newborn babies who are sexually inexperienced has been reported in various studies which suggests plausible non-sexual alternative route of HPV infection. Detection of HPV genotypes and their similarities in the offspring's oral sample and in mother's genital tract suggests that the probable source of HPV infection in the newborn is the HPV infected mother. In the mother-baby pair, the reported vertical transmission rates are between 18.2 and 53.3% [88].

The possible mode of vertical transmission of HPV to infant from a mother is still under debate. However, during fertilization, or pregnancy or delivery the possible mode of transmission has been implicated. Evidence of prenatal transmission of HPV has been provided by Koskimaa et al. [89] and the presence of HPV in cord blood and placenta has been shown to increase the risk of carrying HPV DNA in the oral mucosa which suggests that in the transmission of HPV, unlike several other human viruses, placenta may play an important role [27]. Recent studies reported that the placenta and the maternal microbiomes have role in regulating the neonatal microbiomes which suggests during pregnancy the fetal exposure of microbiota has long-term outcomes in their health [90]. The translocated maternal oral microbes are presented to the fetal immune system at the placenta which acts as a site leading to the development of prenatal tolerance to the maternal microbiome [91].

The encounter with HPV and its significance in pre or perinatal period is not clear. Early exposure of HPV might have a significant impact in the HPV-specific immunity development, subsequent HPV infection and progression due to the immaturity of the immune system of the fetus and infant [92]. However, practically in children the HPV-specific immunity has remained an unknown area. As reported by Koskimaa et al. [88] and Koskimaa et al. [93], children aged 12–14 years had immunoreactivity specific to HPV 16 E2-, E6-, and E7. Whereas, various studies reported that the HPV-16 specific cell mediated immunity is much lower in adults [94, 95]. Between HPV positive and negative subjects, differences have been found in the memory Th cell (T Helper) reactivity against HPV16 E2, E7 and E6 oncoproteins in adults. Against HPV16 E2 and E6, the Th responsiveness is accompanied by the type 1 and type 2 cytokine secretions in a mixed pattern and seems to be more common in healthy individuals as compared to individuals with HPV16 induced disease.

Koskimaa et al. [89] reported that children those are exposed to HPV via cord blood or Oral HPV or placenta might have HPV16 specific T helper cell responses similar to the adults having HPV induced lesions which are highly different from negative HPV controls.

Though some studies have reported HPV infection to be associated with spontaneous preterm delivery and spontaneous abortion, controversy continues in this field due to the reason that some studies were unable to confirm this association.

6. Potential of HPV infection during pregnancy can lead to the development of cervical cancer and therapeutic strategies

Cervical cancer ranks as the 3rd most frequently diagnosed cancer with an estimated 569,847 incident cases and 311,365 deaths reported in the year 2018 (GLOBOCAN) worldwide and in women it is the fourth leading cause of death due to cancer. After breast cancer it ranks second in incidence and mortality rates in lower HDI settings. Worldwide in 28 countries it is the mostly diagnosed cancer and leading cause of cancer death in 42 countries which includes vast majority in South-Eastern Asia and Sub-Saharan Africa [96]. It has been reported that around 530,000 women get affected every year by cervical cancer and the HPV related cancer burden in women worldwide add up to 6% of total cancer cases.

In India, the diagnosis of new cervical cancer is about 96,922 cases annually making it the 2nd leading cause of female cancer. Women aged between 15 and 44 years, cervical cancer is the second most common female cancer in India [97].

The development of cervical cancer and its precursor lesions are reported through several epidemiological and biological studies to be associated with high-risk Human papillomavirus (HPV) infection. The development of high grade cervical lesions is reported to be associated with positive high-risk HPV test results in women with or without abnormal cervical smears [66, 98–100]. It has been reported in various studies on immunocompromised patients such as transplant recipients and AIDs patients that the increased persistence of high-risk HPV and HPV-mediated carcinogenesis is associated with compromised immunosurveillance [101, 102]. In pregnancy, the immune-response is altered in women and some studies concluded that there is no effect of pregnancy on CIN [103], whereas few reported high relapse rates of cervical dysplasia in the postpartum period [104]. Likewise, few studies reported high-risk HPV prevalence rate to be higher in pregnant women and others reported there is no difference of HPV prevalence between non-pregnant and pregnant women. However, on the natural course of high-risk HPV types infection the influence of pregnancy is not yet known. There are few questions need to be answered in this area: (1) what is the difference between the clearance of HPV in pregnant and non-pregnant women? (2) During pregnancy how does the high-risk HPV rate change? [6].

The Food and Drug Administration (FDA) has approved three vaccines such as the first-generation Human papillomavirus (HPV) vaccines, Gardasil (Merck, Kenilworth, NJ, USA) which is a quadri valent vaccine; Cervarix (GlaxoSmithKline, London, UK) which is a bivalent vaccine, have the potential to prevent about 70 and 84% of the cervical cancer cases respectively. Gardasil 9 (Merck), which is a next-generation nonavalent HPV vaccine, can prevent cervical cancer approximately 90%. However, pre-existing infections and their related cervical abnormalities cannot be treated by these vaccines. The American Society of Clinical Oncology (ASCO) in the year 2016 released cervical screening guidelines which recommend the screening for women aged between 30 and 49 years, one to three times in a lifetime in lower resource settings [105]. The screening should be done with primary HPV testing via the use of self-collected specimens as it has been reported to be more effective, adaptable and reliable method of screening as compared to traditional cytological methods and thus the effective cervical cancer screening can be done in several generations of women [106].

In terms of HPV vaccination and coverage rates of cervical screening, considerable inconsistencies exist worldwide between countries and within countries. In low-income and middle-income countries (LMICs), in the year 2008 the reported overall screening uptake was 19%, while in high-income regions it was 63% [107].

As compared to high-income countries, in low-income and middle-income countries the HPV vaccination coverage is much lower. In the high-income countries an estimated 33.6% of girls and women aged between 10 and 20 years had received the full course of HPV vaccine by the year 2014 as compared to low-income and middle-income countries which was 2.7% of the same age group of females [108]. Though studies are still in progress on the long-term vaccine efficacies to understand the total duration of protection, it has been reported that with Gardasil the protection against targeted HPV types last for at least 10 years [109], with Cervarix at least 9 years [110] and with Gardasil 9 a least 6 years [111]. But these vaccines have not sufficiently been tested during pregnancy and hence it is not used in pregnant women.

The Centers for Disease Control and Prevention (CDC) recommends HPV vaccination for women having either an HPV infection or an abnormal Pap test or both if they are in the appropriate age group as that may protect them against the high-risk HPV types which have not been acquired by them. However, the vaccination has not the potential to treat the abnormal results of the Pap test or cure the current HPV infections [112]. Though, the vaccines have been reported to be safe when given to people with pre-existing HPV infection, it gives maximum benefit if given to people before being sexually active [113, 114]. However, some residual benefit from the vaccination will still be there for people already exposed to HPV even though infections with one or more HPV types which are included in the vaccines. Currently, there is no specific test available to detect past exposure of HPV in individuals and the approved HPV tests detect only current infection with high-risk HPV types at the cervix region without any information on past infection.

Even after the vaccination, the screening for cervical cancer need to be done as all HPV types which has the potential to cause cancer are not covered by the HPV vaccines. Therefore, in cervical cells to detect precancerous changes before the development of cancer, screening is essential. Additionally, women with existing HPV infection or who are not vaccinated the cervical screening is critically important. However, the screening recommendations may be changed in future for women given HPV vaccination.

Research works are in progress to develop therapeutic HPV vaccines which would prevent cancer development among women with previous history of HPV infection. The immune system will be stimulated by these vaccines which will result in specifically targeting and killing infected cells. The safety and efficacy of a therapeutic DNA vaccine are being tested by ongoing clinical trials to treat HPV related cervical and vulvar lesions [115–117]. A combination of preventive and therapeutic vaccine would be an ideal strategy in this case.

Topical microbicides is another preventive strategy which is being explored. In various studies, carrageenan which is an extracted compound from seaweed widely used in foods and other products has been reported to inhibit infection with HPV. Clinical trial in healthy individuals with a gel containing carrageenan is underway to test its efficacy to prevent genital HPV infections.

6.1 Immunization of the pregnant women

The response of the adaptive immune system of the infants cannot be protective to many pathogens in the first months of life. The T cells of both fetal and neonatal origin are shewed towards Th2 responses which are ineffective against intracellular pathogens. Ineffectiveness has also been reported for bacterial polysaccharides by antibody responses. Infants rely on additional protection during this period which is acquired from maternal antibodies during gestation passively transported through the placenta. At the time of birth, the antibody levels present in the infants are correlated with the maternal antibody levels and the therefore, there is an interconnection between the antibody levels present in the maternal circulation and the degree of transfer of antibodies. However, the suboptimal maternal specific antibodies may not be sufficient to provide full protective immunity or can provide protection only for a limited period of time to the infants. Moreover, the maternal antibody levels decrease over a periods of approximately 6 months after birth. Therefore, the aim of the maternal immunization is to increase the concentration of maternal specific antibody and their passive transport to the fetus which will reduce the window of vulnerability for infants. IgG (Immunoglobulin G) is the only isotype among the five antibody classes that has the ability to efficiently cross the human placenta. Syncytiotrophoblast cells of the placenta, are responsible for the transfer of the IgG antibodies from mother to the fetus, which are located in contact with the maternal blood. In the circulation maternal IgG are internalized in endosomes and bind to Fc receptors (FcRn) of the neonatal cells which are expressed on the surface of the internal endosomes. On membrane of the fetal side of the syncytiotrophoblasts, the endosomes fuse and the IgG are released from FcRn. Passing through the villous stroma and fetal capillary endothelium, IgG enters the fetal circulation through an unknown mechanism. With the largest transferred proportion during the third trimester of pregnancy, the transfer of IgG through placenta increases over time especially within the last 4 weeks. Consistent with an active transport process, the IgG concentration in the fetal circulation are generally greater than the maternal circulation at full term of pregnancy [118, 119]. This transfer is influenced by several factors such as maternal non-infectious diseases, placental integrity, total maternal IgG concentration, FcRn availability, IgG subtype, timing of infection or vaccination and nature of the antigen [120]. IgG4, IgG3 and IgG2 are the least efficiently transferred to the fetus as compared to IgG1 which is the most efficiently transferred antibody subtype to the fetus.

Approximately after 2 weeks of maternal immunization, the concentration of specific antibodies starts increasing which suggests that if the vaccination is provided between 28 and 32 weeks of pregnancy, the optimal amount of specific IgG may be achieved in full-term infants at birth, but may not be the same for preterm infants. Diphtheria toxoid-acellular pertussis vaccine (Tdap) in the second trimester is reported to be reduced by the vaccination with tetanus toxoid which results in higher neonatal anti-pertussis antibody titers as compared to vaccination in the third trimester both in preterm and term neonates [121, 122]. The total longer transfer time may be a reason for the accumulation of antibodies in the fetal circulation. In addition to the maternal IgG antibodies which is transferred through placenta and known for providing protection, lesser concentration of IgG, IgM and high concentration of maternal IgA are also excreted in the breast milk and colostrum [123]. Immediately after delivery or in the second or third trimester of pregnancy, vaccination with Tdap reported to increase the pertussis-specific IgA antibody levels in the breast milk [124]. Therefore, another mode of transferring antibodies to the new born is breastfeeding. The maternal IgA transferred through the breast milk helps protecting the infants against enteric infections and respiratory illness with fever in infants born to influenza-vaccinated mothers for at least 6 months after birth [42, 123]. Though, there are evidences highlighting the maternal immunization benefits, few studies have also shown controversial interferences between the maternal IgG antibodies and the infant antibody responses [125].

The "immunological blunting", a phenomenon is observed after the primary vaccination series in early infancy when the maternal IgG antibodies can inhibit the immune responses against the same or related antigens. While after the booster dose, this blunting effect dissipates [119, 126]. Blunting has been reported to be observed with polio and measles vaccines after natural infection or maternal immunization for maternal antibodies [119, 127]. Though, the clinical importance of this blunting effect is unknown, the epidemiological data of implemented maternal immunization from various countries have not shown any negative impact on the protection against the diseases targeted [26, 128].

6.2 HPV vaccination during pregnancy

Gardasil and Cervarix both HPV vaccines are recombinant which contains virus-like particles (VLP's) and enhanced by an adjuvant which is responsible for triggering an immune response higher than a natural infection [129]. Gardasil 9, a 9-valent HPV vaccine was only licensed for use in the USA in December 2014.

Depending on age, full coverage by the HPV vaccine is obtained by 2 or 3 doses with the first dose administered at time o, followed by the second dose after 1–2 months and the third dose after 6 months [130]. While, all doses are not received by many girls [131]. In order to achieve long-term duration of immunity, the repeat doses of vaccine are given which boost the immune system.

Worldwide, millions of doses of HPV vaccine since its introduction have been administered and involuntary administration also occurs during pregnancy as the young fertile women are the main recipients of the vaccines. Potentially harmful adverse effects (AE) to the unborn child such as preterm birth, miscarriage, congenital malformations, fetal death or fears of teratogenicity raise concern among both the health care providers and recipients. The development of sensitive organs such as the heart, the central nervous system takes place in the first trimester of pregnancy and in this period the environmental factors like medications and drugs theoretically might cause damage the developing fetus which is the main reason of concern. The vaccine manufacturers (Merck and GlaxoSmithKline) and the World Health Organization recommend avoiding HPV vaccination during pregnancy [36]. However, in case of accidental vaccination of pregnant women there are no interventions and no mandatory pregnancy testing before vaccination recommended so far. Moreover, conducting studies to investigate the pregnancy outcomes by administering HPV vaccines to pregnant women are not ethically feasible. In pregnancy, the true safety of the HPV vaccination has not yet been established through randomized controlled trial. Hence, the HPV vaccine administration to the pregnant women has not yet been approved [132].

7. Conclusion

In pregnant women, many observational studies reported the HPV infection risk but there are controversial results too. Higher HPV prevalence has been reported in few studies, whereas several studies reported lower prevalence in pregnant women or there is no statistical difference between pregnant and age matched non-pregnant controls [16].

For a successful pregnancy, a modulated, dynamic and responsive immune system is required but definitely not a suppressive one and this has been supported by an increasing number of studies. At the feto-maternal interface, the trophoblastic cells are important for the receptive immune system establishment which is achieved as a part of response mechanism to the normal microbiota which highlights the complexity of the regulatory pathways involved during pregnancy. Moreover, there are evidences on the effects that changed the modulated immune system and the receptive feto-maternal interface by a clinically silent viral infection emphasizes the necessity of better detection, treatment and prevention of the viral infections during pregnancy. This will further lead not only to the better outcomes of pregnancy but also the postnatal development can be affected in a better way as these viral infections and the subsequent inflammations reported to be associated with mental health issues and diseases of the immune system such as asthma and allergies. The effects of viral infections on fetal development during pregnancy can more be exemplified by the recent Zika virus outbreak and its teratogenic effect on the development of brain [22]. Therefore, it is important to understand the complex immune responses during pregnancy, with the continued risk of pandemics and the emergence of newer diseases associated as secondary to the viral infection, which will lead to the development of appropriate approaches and tools to protect both the fetus and the mother [41].

Moreover, there are very limited data is available due to the very limited number of investigations have been performed on materials from spontaneous abortions and spontaneous preterm deliveries due to HPV infection and the heterogeneous study groups making it difficult to come to a reliable conclusion. A proper study design, selection of proper controls is very essential in this case and a strict control of the similarity in patients/samples is needed for a valuable comparison between studies. Furthermore, the simple detection of a virus cannot be a real causative role for diseases in general or adverse pregnancy outcomes. Therefore, for this particular situation it is important to study the cellular localization and the viral activity to come to a realistic conclusion.

Therefore, we recommend more investigations on materials of adverse pregnancy outcomes including spontaneous abortion and spontaneous preterm delivery and the molecular mechanism of HPV infections on it which is the need of the hour and researchers need to conduct new studies to clarify the exact molecular mechanisms involved on the HPV infection in early pregnancy and how the self-clearance takes place during the course of pregnancy.

Conflict of interest

The authors declare no conflict of interest.

Author details

Sanchita Roy Pradhan, Sutapa Mahata, Dipanwita Ghosh, Pranab Kumar Sahoo, Sinjini Sarkar, Ranita Pal and Vilas D. Nasare*
Department of Pathology and Cancer Screening, Chittaranjan National Cancer Institute, Kolkata, India

*Address all correspondence to: vilas.dr@gmail.com

References

[1] Trottier H, Mayrand MH, Baggio ML, Galan L, Ferenczy A, Villa LL, et al. Ludwig-McGill cohort study group. Risk of human papillomavirus (HPV) infection and cervical Neoplasia after pregnancy. BMC Pregnancy and Childbirth. 2015;**15**:244. DOI: 10.1186/s12884-015-0675-0

[2] Mor G. Placental inflammatory response to Zika virus may affect fetal brain development. American Journal of Reproductive Immunology. 2016;**75**(4):421-422. DOI: 10.1111/aji.12505

[3] Laskarin G, Kämmerer U, Rukavina D, Thomson AW, Fernandez N, Blois SM. Antigen-presenting cells and materno-fetal tolerance: An emerging role for dendritic cells. American Journal of Reproductive Immunology. 2007;**58**(3):255-267

[4] Moffett-King A. Natural killer cells and pregnancy. Nature Reviews Immunology. 2002;**2**(9):656-663. Review. Erratum in: Nature Reviews Immunology. 2002;**2**(12):975

[5] Hanna J, Goldman-Wohl D, Hamani Y, Avraham I, Greenfield C, Natanson-Yaron S, et al. Decidual NK cells regulate key developmental processes at the human fetal-maternal interface. Nature Medicine. 2006;**12**(9):1065-1074

[6] Nobbenhuis MA, Helmerhorst TJ, van den Brule AJ, Rozendaal L, Bezemer PD, Voorhorst FJ, et al. High-risk human papillomavirus clearance in pregnant women: Trends for lower clearance during pregnancy with a catch-up postpartum. British Journal of Cancer. 2002;**87**(1):75-80

[7] Jalil EM, Bastos FI, Melli PP, Duarte G, Simoes RT, Yamamoto AY, et al. HPV clearance in postpartum period of HIV-positive and negative women: A prospective follow-up study. BMC Infectious Diseases. 2013;**13**:564. DOI: 10.1186/1471-2334-13-564

[8] Michelin D, Gissmann L, Street D, Potkul RK, Fisher S, Kaufmann AM, et al. Regulation of human papillomavirus type 18 in vivo: Effects of estrogen and progesterone in transgenic mice. Gynecologic Oncology. 1997;**66**(2):202-208

[9] Yamasaki K, Miura K, Shimada T, Miura S, Abe S, Murakami M, et al. Epidemiology of human papillomavirus genotypes in pregnant Japanese women. Journal of Human Genetics. 2011;**56**(4):313-315. DOI: 10.1038/jhg.2011.11

[10] Michaeli TF, Bergman Y, Gielchinsky Y. Rejuvenating effect of pregnancy on the mother. Fertility and Sterility. 2015;**103**(5):1125-1128

[11] Bosch FX, Burchell AN, Schiffman M, Giuliano AR, de Sanjose S, Bruni L, et al. Epidemiology and natural history of human papillomavirus infections and type-specific implications in cervical neoplasia. Vaccine. 2008;**26**(Suppl 10):K1-K16. DOI: 10.1016/j.vaccine.2008.05.064

[12] Trottier H, Burchell AN. Epidemiology of mucosal human papillomavirus infection and associated diseases. Public Health Genomics. 2009;**12**(5-6):291-307. DOI: 10.1159/000214920

[13] Bruni L, Diaz M, Castellsagué X, Ferrer E, Bosch FX, de Sanjosé S. Cervical human papillomavirus prevalence in 5 continents: Meta-analysis of 1 million women with normal cytological findings. The Journal of Infectious Diseases. 2010;**202**(12):1789-1799. DOI: 10.1086/657321

[14] Trottier H, Ferreira S, Thomann P, Costa MC, Sobrinho JS, Prado JC, et al. Human papillomavirus infection and reinfection in adult women: The role of sexual activity and natural immunity. Cancer Research. 2010;**70**(21):8569-8577. DOI: 10.1158/0008-5472.CAN-10-0621

[15] Skinner SR, Wheeler CM, Romanowski B, Castellsagué X, Lazcano-Ponce E, Del Rosario-Raymundo MR, et al. Progression of HPV infection to detectable cervical lesions or clearance in adult women: Analysis of the control arm of the VIVIANE study. The International Journal of Cancer. 2016;**138**(10):2428-2438. DOI: 10.1002/ijc.29971

[16] Liu P, Xu L, Sun Y, Wang Z. The prevalence and risk of human papillomavirus infection in pregnant women. Epidemiology and Infection. 2014;**142**(8):1567-1578. DOI: 10.1017/S0950268814000636

[17] Castellsagué X, Drudis T, Cañadas MP, Goncé A, Ros R, Pérez JM, et al. Human papillomavirus (HPV) infection in pregnant women and mother-to-child transmission of genital HPV genotypes: A prospective study in Spain. BMC Infectious Diseases. 2009;**9**:74. DOI: 10.1186/1471-2334-9-74

[18] Niyibizi J, Zanré N, Mayrand MH, Trottier H. The association between adverse pregnancy outcomes and maternal human papillomavirus infection: A systematic review protocol. Systematic Reviews. 2017;**6**(1):53. DOI: 10.1186/s13643-017-0443-5

[19] de Sanjosé S, Diaz M, Castellsagué X, Clifford G, Bruni L, Muñoz N, et al. Worldwide prevalence and genotype distribution of cervical human papillomavirus DNA in women with normal cytology: A meta-analysis. The Lancet Infectious Diseases. 2007;**7**(7):453-459

[20] Pandey D, Solleti V, Jain G, Das A, Shama Prasada K, Acharya S, et al. Human papillomavirus (HPV) infection in early pregnancy: Prevalence and implications. Infectious Diseases in Obstetrics and Gynecology. 2019;**2019**:4376902. DOI: 10.1155/2019/4376902

[21] Gloss B, Bernard HU, Seedorf K, Klock G. The upstream regulatory region of the human papilloma virus-16 contains an E2 protein-independent enhancer which is specific for cervical carcinoma cells and regulated by glucocorticoid hormones. The EMBO Journal. 1987;**6**(12):3735-3743

[22] Mor G, Cardenas I. The immune system in pregnancy: A unique complexity. American Journal of Reproductive Immunology. 2010;**63**(6):425-433. DOI: 10.1111/j.1600-0897.2010.00836.x

[23] Gellersen B, Brosens IA, Brosens JJ. Decidualization of the human endometrium: Mechanisms, functions, and clinical perspectives. Seminars in Reproductive Medicine. 2007;**25**(6):445-453

[24] Chaouat G, Petitbarat M, Dubanchet S, Rahmati M, Ledée N. Tolerance to the foetal allograft? American Journal of Reproductive Immunology. 2010;**63**(6):624-636. DOI: 10.1111/j.1600-0897.2010.00832.x

[25] Omer SB. Maternal immunization. The New England Journal of Medicine. 2017;**376**(13):1256-1267. DOI: 10.1056/NEJMra1509044

[26] Vojtek I, Dieussaert I, Doherty TM, Franck V, Hanssens L, Miller J, et al. Maternal immunization: Where are we now and how to move forward? Annals of Medicine. 2018;**50**(3):193-208. DOI: 10.1080/07853890.2017.1421320

[27] Younes AS, Csire M, Kapusinszky B, Szomor K, Takács M, Berencsi G.

Heterogeneous pathways of maternal-fetal transmission of human viruses (review). Pathology Oncology Research. 2009;**15**(3):451-465. DOI: 10.1007/s12253-009-9166-9

[28] You H, Liu Y, Agrawal N, Prasad CK, Chiriva-Internati M, Lowery CL, et al. Infection, replication, and cytopathology of human papillomavirus type 31 in trophoblasts. Virology. 2003;**316**(2):281-289

[29] Freitas AC, Mariz FC, Silva MA, Jesus AL. Human papillomavirus vertical transmission: Review of current data. Clinical Infectious Diseases. 2013;**56**(10):1451-1456. DOI: 10.1093/cid/cit066

[30] Croy BA, van den Heuvel MJ, Borzychowski AM, Tayade C. Uterine natural killer cells: A specialized differentiation regulated by ovarian hormones. Immunological Reviews. 2006;**214**:161-185

[31] Gomez LM, Ma Y, Ho C, McGrath CM, Nelson DB, Parry S. Placental infection with human papillomavirus is associated with spontaneous preterm delivery. Human Reproduction. 2008;**23**(3):709-715. DOI: 10.1093/humrep/dem404

[32] Ramhorst R, Fraccaroli L, Aldo P, Alvero AB, Cardenas I, Leirós CP, et al. Modulation and recruitment of inducible regulatory T cells by first trimester trophoblast cells. American Journal of Reproductive Immunology. 2012;**67**(1):17-27. DOI: 10.1111/j.1600-0897.2011.01056.x. Epub Aug 7, 2011

[33] Manaster I, Mizrahi S, Goldman-Wohl D, Sela HY, Stern-Ginossar N, Lankry D, et al. Endometrial NK cells are special immature cells that await pregnancy. Journal of Immunology. 2008;**181**(3):1869-1876

[34] Zhang J, Chen Z, Smith GN, Croy BA. Natural killer cell-triggered vascular transformation: Maternal care before birth? Cellular and Molecular Immunology. 2011;**8**(1):1-11. DOI: 10.1038/cmi.2010.38

[35] Houser BL, Tilburgs T, Hill J, Nicotra ML, Strominger JL. Two unique human decidual macrophage populations. Journal of Immunology. 2011;**186**(4):2633-2642. DOI: 10.4049/jimmunol.1003153

[36] Pregnancy Guidelines and Recommendations by Vaccine | CDC [Internet]. Centers for Disease Control and Prevention. Centers for Disease Control and Prevention. Available from: https://www.cdc.gov/vaccines/pregnancy/hcp-toolkit/guidelines.html?CDC_AA_refVal=https://www.cdc.gov/vaccines/pregnancy/hcp/guidelines.html [Cited Oct 10, 2019]

[37] Lockwood CJ, Huang SJ, Chen CP, Huang Y, Xu J, Faramarzi S, et al. Decidual cell regulation of natural killer cell-recruiting chemokines: Implications for the pathogenesis and prediction of preeclampsia. The American Journal of Pathology. 2013;**183**(3):841-856. DOI: 10.1016/j.ajpath.2013.05.029

[38] Nancy P, Tagliani E, Tay CS, Asp P, Levy DE, Erlebacher A. Chemokine gene silencing in decidual stromal cells limits T cell access to the maternal-fetal interface. Science. 2012;**336**(6086):1317-1321. DOI: 10.1126/science.1220030

[39] Abrahams VM, Visintin I, Aldo PB, Guller S, Romero R, Mor G. A role for TLRs in the regulation of immune cell migration by first trimester trophoblast cells. Journal of Immunology. 2005;**175**(12):8096-8104

[40] Costello MJ, Joyce SK, Abrahams VM. NOD protein expression and function in first trimester trophoblast cells. American Journal of Reproductive Immunology. 2007;**57**(1):67-80

[41] Mor G, Aldo P, Alvero AB. The unique immunological and microbial aspects of pregnancy. Nature Reviews. Immunology. 2017;**17**(8):469-482. DOI: 10.1038/nri.2017.64

[42] Silasi M, Cardenas I, Kwon JY, Racicot K, Aldo P, Mor G. Viral infections during pregnancy. American Journal of Reproductive Immunology. 2015;**73**(3):199-213. DOI: 10.1111/aji.12355

[43] Coyne CB, Lazear HM. Zika virus—reigniting the TORCH. Nature Reviews. Microbiology. 2016;**14**(11):707-715. DOI: 10.1038/nrmicro.2016.125

[44] Giugliano S, Petroff MG, Warren BD, Jasti S, Linscheid C, Ward A, et al. Hepatitis C virus sensing by human Trophoblasts induces innate immune responses and recruitment of maternal NK cells: Potential implications for limiting vertical transmission. Journal of Immunology. 2015;**195**(8):3737-3747. DOI: 10.4049/jimmunol.1500409

[45] Tian M, Zhang Y, Liu Z, Sun G, Mor G, Liao A. The PD-1/PD-L1 inhibitory pathway is altered in pre-eclampsia and regulates T cell responses in pre-eclamptic rats. Scientific Reports. 2016;**6**:27683. DOI: 10.1038/srep27683

[46] Olivadoti M, Toth LA, Weinberg J, Opp MR. Murine gammaherpesvirus 68: A model for the study of Epstein-Barr virus infections and related diseases. Comparative Medicine. 2007;**57**(1):44-50

[47] Racicot K, Kwon JY, Aldo P, Abrahams V, El-Guindy A, Romero R, et al. Type I interferon regulates the placental inflammatory response to bacteria and is targeted by virus: Mechanism of polymicrobial infection-induced preterm birth. American Journal of Reproductive Immunology. 2016;**75**(4):451-460. DOI: 10.1111/aji.12501

[48] Cardenas I, Means RE, Aldo P, Koga K, Lang SM, Booth CJ, et al. Viral infection of the placenta leads to fetal inflammation and sensitization to bacterial products predisposing to preterm labor. Journal of Immunology. 2010;**185**(2):1248-1257. DOI: 10.4049/jimmunol.1000289

[49] Cappelletti M, Presicce P, Lawson MJ, Chaturvedi V, Stankiewicz TE, Vanoni S, et al. Type I interferons regulate susceptibility to inflammation-induced preterm birth. JCI Insight. 2017;**2**(5):e91288. DOI: 10.1172/jci.insight.91288

[50] Lapaire O, Holzgreve W, Oosterwijk JC, Brinkhaus R, Bianchi DW. Georg Schmorl on trophoblasts in the maternal circulation. Placenta. 2007;**28**(1):1-5. Epub Apr 18, 2006

[51] Bianchi DW, Zickwolf GK, Weil GJ, Sylvester S, DeMaria MA. Male fetal progenitor cells persist in maternal blood for as long as 27 years postpartum. Proceedings of the National Academy of Sciences of the United States of America. 1996;**93**(2):705-708

[52] O'Donoghue K, Chan J, de la Fuente J, Kennea N, Sandison A, Anderson JR, et al. Microchimerism in female bone marrow and bone decades after fetal mesenchymal stem-cell trafficking in pregnancy. Lancet. 2004;**364**(9429):179-182

[53] Koopmans M, Kremer Hovinga IC, Baelde HJ, Fernandes RJ, de Heer E, Bruijn JA, et al. Chimerism in kidneys, livers and hearts of normal women: Implications for transplantation studies. American Journal of Transplantation. 2005;**5**(6):1495-1502

[54] Desai RG, Creger WP. Maternofetal passage of leukocytes and platelets in man. Blood. 1963;**21**:665-673

[55] Maloney S, Smith A, Furst DE, Myerson D, Rupert K, Evans PC, et al.

Microchimerism of maternal origin persists into adult life. The Journal of Clinical Investigation. 1999;**104**(1):41-47

[56] Ariga H, Ohto H, Busch MP, Imamura S, Watson R, Reed W, et al. Kinetics of fetal cellular and cell-free DNA in the maternal circulation during and after pregnancy: Implications for noninvasive prenatal diagnosis. Transfusion. 2001;**41**(12):1524-1530

[57] Lo YM, Lo ES, Watson N, Noakes L, Sargent IL, Thilaganathan B, et al. Two-way cell traffic between mother and fetus: Biologic and clinical implications. Blood. 1996;**88**(11):4390-4395

[58] Jeanty C, Derderian SC, Mackenzie TC. Maternal-fetal cellular trafficking: Clinical implications and consequences. Current Opinion in Pediatrics. 2014;**26**(3):377-382. DOI: 10.1097/MOP.0000000000000087

[59] Yan Z, Lambert NC, Guthrie KA, Porter AJ, Loubiere LS, Madeleine MM, et al. Male microchimerism in women without sons: Quantitative assessment and correlation with pregnancy history. The American Journal of Medicine. 2005;**118**(8):899-906

[60] Tanaka A, Lindor K, Ansari A, Gershwin ME. Fetal microchimerisms in the mother: Immunologic implications. Liver Transplantation. 2000;**6**(2):138-143

[61] Bianchi DW, Fisk NM. Fetomaternal cell trafficking and the stem cell debate: Gender matters. Journal of the American Medical Association. 2007;**297**(13):1489-1491

[62] Knippen MA. Microchimerism: Sharing genes in illness and in health. ISRN Nursing. 2011;**2011**:893819. DOI: 10.5402/2011/893819

[63] Chen CP, Lee MY, Huang JP, Aplin JD, Wu YH, Hu CS, et al. Trafficking of multipotent mesenchymal stromal cells from maternal circulation through the placenta involves vascular endothelial growth factor receptor-1 and integrins. Stem Cells. 2008;**26**(2):550-561

[64] Berry SM, Hassan SS, Russell E, Kukuruga D, Land S, Kaplan J. Association of maternal histocompatibility at class II HLA loci with maternal microchimerism in the fetus. Pediatric Research. 2004;**56**(1):73-78

[65] Lambert NC, Evans PC, Hashizumi TL, Maloney S, Gooley T, Furst DE, et al. Cutting edge: Persistent fetal microchimerism in T lymphocytes is associated with HLA-DQA1*0501: Implications in autoimmunity. Journal of Immunology. 2000;**164**(11):5545-5548

[66] Rozendaal L, Walboomers JM, van der Linden JC, Voorhorst FJ, Kenemans P, Helmerhorst TJ, et al. PCR-based high-risk HPV test in cervical cancer screening gives objective risk assessment of women with cytomorphologically normal cervical smears. International Journal of Cancer. 1996;**68**(6):766-769

[67] Khosrotehrani K, Guegan S, Fraitag S, Oster M, de Prost Y, Bodemer C, et al. Presence of chimeric maternally derived keratinocytes in cutaneous inflammatory diseases of children: The example of pityriasis lichenoides. The Journal of Investigative Dermatology. 2006;**126**(2):345-348

[68] Khosrotehrani K, Johnson KL, Cha DH, Salomon RN, Bianchi DW. Transfer of fetal cells with multilineage potential to maternal tissue. Journal of the American Medical Association. 2004;**292**(1):75-80

[69] Stevens AM, Hermes HM, Rutledge JC, Buyon JP, Nelson JL. Myocardial-tissue-specific phenotype of

maternal microchimerism in neonatal lupus congenital heart block. Lancet. 2003;**362**(9396):1617-1623

[70] Vanzyl B, Planas R, Ye Y, Foulis A, de Krijger RR, Vives-Pi M, et al. Why are levels of maternal microchimerism higher in type 1 diabetes pancreas? Chimerism. 2010;**1**(2):45-50. DOI: 10.4161/chim.1.2.13891

[71] Mold JE, Michaëlsson J, Burt TD, Muench MO, Beckerman KP, Busch MP, et al. Maternal alloantigens promote the development of tolerogenic fetal regulatory T cells in utero. Science. 2008;**322**(5907):1562-1565. DOI: 10.1126/science.1164511

[72] Gadi VK, Nelson JL. Fetal microchimerism in women with breast cancer. Cancer Research. 2007;**67**(19):9035-9038

[73] Cirello V, Perrino M, Colombo C, Muzza M, Filopanti M, Vicentini L, et al. Fetal cell microchimerism in papillary thyroid cancer: Studies in peripheral blood and tissues. International Journal of Cancer. 2010;**126**(12):2874-2878. DOI: 10.1002/ijc.24993

[74] Dutta P, Molitor-Dart M, Bobadilla JL, Roenneburg DA, Yan Z, Torrealba JR, et al. Microchimerism is strongly correlated with tolerance to noninherited maternal antigens in mice. Blood. 2009;**114**(17):3578-3587. DOI: 10.1182/blood-2009-03-213561

[75] Opiela SJ, Levy RB, Adkins B. Murine neonates develop vigorous in vivo cytotoxic and Th1/Th2 responses upon exposure to low doses of NIMA-like alloantigens. Blood. 2008;**112**(4):1530-1538. DOI: 10.1182/blood-2007-08-106500

[76] Farina A, Sekizawa A, Sugito Y, Iwasaki M, Jimbo M, Saito H, et al. Fetal DNA in maternal plasma as a screening variable for preeclampsia. A preliminary nonparametric analysis of detection rate in low-risk nonsymptomatic patients. Prenatal Diagnosis. 2004;**24**(2):83-86

[77] Jakobsen TR, Clausen FB, Rode L, Dziegiel MH, Tabor A. High levels of fetal DNA are associated with increased risk of spontaneous preterm delivery. Prenatal Diagnosis. 2012;**32**(9):840-845. DOI: 10.1002/pd.3917

[78] Rava RP, Srinivasan A, Sehnert AJ, Bianchi DW. Circulating fetal cell-free DNA fractions differ in autosomal aneuploidies and monosomy X. Clinical Chemistry. 2014;**60**(1):243-250. DOI: 10.1373/clinchem.2013.207951

[79] Merckx M et al. Transmission of carcinogenic human papillomavirus types from mother to child: A metaanalysis of published studies. European Journal of Cancer Prevention. 2012

[80] Koullali B, Oudijk MA, Nijman TA, Mol BW, Pajkrt E. Risk assessment and management to prevent preterm birth. Seminars in Fetal and Neonatal Medicine. 2016;**21**(2):80-88. DOI: 10.1016/j.siny.2016.01.005

[81] Ambühl LM, Baandrup U, Dybkær K, Blaakær J, Uldbjerg N, Sørensen S. Human papillomavirus infection as a possible cause of spontaneous abortion and spontaneous preterm delivery. Infectious Diseases in Obstetrics and Gynecology. 2016;**2016**:3086036. DOI: 10.1155/2016/3086036

[82] Barker DJ. Fetal origins of coronary heart disease. BMJ. 1995;**311**(6998):171-174

[83] Barker DJP. Fetal and infant origins of adult disease. Monatsschrift Kinderheilkunde. 2001;**149**(Suppl. 1): S2-S6. DOI: 10.1007/s001120170002

[84] Bateson P, Barker D, Clutton-Brock T, Deb D, D'Udine B, Foley RA, et al. Developmental plasticity

and human health. Nature. 2004;**430**(6998):419-421

[85] Hales CN, Barker DJ. The thrifty phenotype hypothesis. British Medical Bulletin. 2001;**60**:5-20

[86] Ben-Shlomo Y, Kuh D. A life course approach to chronic disease epidemiology: Conceptual models, empirical challenges and interdisciplinary perspectives. International Journal of Epidemiology. 2002;**31**(2):285-293

[87] Skogen JC, Overland S. The fetal origins of adult disease: A narrative review of the epidemiological literature. JRSM Short Reports. 2012;**3**(8):59. DOI: 10.1258/shorts.2012.012048

[88] Koskimaa HM, Paaso A, Welters MJ, Grénman S, Syrjänen K, van der Burg SH, et al. Human papillomavirus 16-specific cell-mediated immunity in children born to mothers with incident cervical intraepithelial neoplasia (CIN) and to those constantly HPV negative. Journal of Translational Medicine. 2015;**13**:370. DOI: 10.1186/s12967-015-0733-4

[89] Koskimaa HM, Paaso A, Welters MJP, Grénman S, Syrjänen K, van der Burg SH, et al. The presence of human papillomavirus (HPV) in placenta and/or cord blood might result in Th2 polarization. European Journal of Clinical Microbiology & Infectious Diseases. 2017;**36**(8):1491-1503. DOI: 10.1007/s10096-017-2958-z

[90] Solt I. The human microbiome and the great obstetrical syndromes: A new frontier in maternal-fetal medicine. Best Practice & Research. Clinical Obstetrics and Gynaecology. 2015;**29**(2):165-175. DOI: 10.1016/j.bpobgyn.2014.04.024

[91] Zaura E, Nicu EA, Krom BP, Keijser BJ. Acquiring and maintaining a normal oral microbiome: Current perspective. Frontiers in Cellular and Infection Microbiology. 2014;**4**:85. DOI: 10.3389/fcimb.2014.00085

[92] Gollwitzer ES, Marsland BJ. Impact of early-life exposures on immune maturation and susceptibility to disease. Trends in Immunology. 2015;**36**(11):684-696. DOI: 10.1016/j.it.2015.09.009

[93] Koskimaa HM, Paaso AE, Welters MJ, Grénman SE, Syrjänen KJ, van der Burg SH, et al. Human papillomavirus 16 E2-, E6- and E7-specific T-cell responses in children and their mothers who developed incident cervical intraepithelial neoplasia during a 14-year follow-up of the Finnish family HPV cohort. Journal of Translational Medicine. 2014;**12**:44. DOI: 10.1186/1479-5876-12-44

[94] Welters MJ, van der Logt P, van den Eeden SJ, Kwappenberg KM, Drijfhout JW, Fleuren GJ, et al. Detection of human papillomavirus type 18 E6 and E7-specific CD4+ T-helper 1 immunity in relation to health versus disease. International Journal of Cancer. 2006;**118**(4):950-956

[95] Woo YL, van den Hende M, Sterling JC, Coleman N, Crawford RA, Kwappenberg KM, et al. A prospective study on the natural course of low-grade squamous intraepithelial lesions and the presence of HPV16 E2-, E6- and E7-specific T-cell responses. International Journal of Cancer. 2010;**126**(1):133-141. DOI: 10.1002/ijc.24804

[96] Bray F, Ferlay J, Soerjomataram I, Siegel RL, Torre LA, Jemal A. Global cancer statistics 2018: GLOBOCAN estimates of incidence and mortality worldwide for 36 cancers in 185 countries. CA: A Cancer Journal for Clinicians. 2018;**68**(6):394-424. DOI: 10.3322/caac.21492

[97] Bruni L, Albero G, Serrano B, Mena M, Gómez D, Muñoz J, Bosch FX,

de Sanjosé S. ICO/IARC Information Centre on HPV and Cancer (HPV Information Centre). Human Papillomavirus and Related Diseases in the World. Summary Report 17 June 2019 [Accessed: Sep 15, 2019]

[98] Ho GY, Burk RD, Klein S, Kadish AS, Chang CJ, Palan P, et al. Persistent genital human papillomavirus infection as a risk factor for persistent cervical dysplasia. Journal of the National Cancer Institute. 1995;**87**(18):1365-1371

[99] Nobbenhuis MA, Walboomers JM, Helmerhorst TJ, Rozendaal L, Remmink AJ, Risse EK, et al. Relation of human papillomavirus status to cervical lesions and consequences for cervical-cancer screening: A prospective study. Lancet. 1999;**354**(9172):20-25. Erratum in: Lancet. 2015;**386**(10002):1446

[100] Remmink AJ, Walboomers JM, Helmerhorst TJ, Voorhorst FJ, Rozendaal L, Risse EK, et al. The presence of persistent high-risk HPV genotypes in dysplastic cervical lesions is associated with progressive disease: Natural history up to 36 months. International Journal of Cancer. 1995;**61**(3):306-311

[101] Petry KU, Köchel H, Bode U, Schedel I, Niesert S, Glaubitz M, et al. Human papillomavirus is associated with the frequent detection of warty and basaloid high-grade neoplasia of the vulva and cervical neoplasia among immunocompromised women. Gynecologic Oncology. 1996;**60**(1):30-34

[102] Sun XW, Kuhn L, Ellerbrock TV, Chiasson MA, Bush TJ, Wright TC Jr. Human papillomavirus infection in women infected with the human immunodeficiency virus. The New England Journal of Medicine. 1997;**337**(19):1343-1349

[103] Jain AG, Higgins RV, Boyle MJ. Management of low-grade squamous intraepithelial lesions during pregnancy. American Journal of Obstetrics and Gynecology. 1997;**177**(2):298-302

[104] Yost NP, Santoso JT, McIntire DD, Iliya FA. Postpartum regression rates of antepartum cervical intraepithelial neoplasia II and III lesions. Obstetrics and Gynecology. 1999;**93**(3):359-362

[105] Jeronimo J, Castle PE, Temin S, Denny L, Gupta V, Kim JJ, et al. Secondary prevention of cervical cancer: ASCO resource-stratified clinical practice guideline. Journal of Global Oncology. 2016;**3**(5):635-657. DOI: 10.1200/JGO.2016.006577

[106] Simms KT, Steinberg J, Caruana M, Smith MA, Lew JB, Soerjomataram I, et al. Impact of scaled up human papillomavirus vaccination and cervical screening and the potential for global elimination of cervical cancer in 181 countries, 2020-99: A modelling study. The Lancet Oncology. 2019;**20**(3):394-407. DOI: 10.1016/S1470-2045(18)30836-2

[107] Gakidou E, Nordhagen S, Obermeyer Z. Coverage of cervical cancer screening in 57 countries: Low average levels and large inequalities. PLoS Medicine. 2008;**5**(6):e132. DOI: 10.1371/journal.pmed.0050132

[108] Bruni L, Diaz M, Barrionuevo-Rosas L, Herrero R, Bray F, Bosch FX, et al. Global estimates of human papillomavirus vaccination coverage by region and income level: A pooled analysis. The Lancet Global Health. 2016;**4**(7):e453-e463. DOI: 10.1016/S2214-109X(16)30099-7. Erratum in: The Lancet Global Health. 2017;**5**(7):e662

[109] Kjaer SK, Nygård M, Dillner J, Brooke Marshall J, Radley D, Li M et al. A 12-year follow-up on the long-term effectiveness of the Quadrivalent human papillomavirus vaccine in 4 Nordic countries. Clinical Infectious

Diseases. 2018;**66**(3):339-345. DOI: 10.1093/cid/cix797

[110] Naud PS, Roteli-Martins CM, De Carvalho NS, Teixeira JC, de Borba PC, Sanchez N, et al. Sustained efficacy, immunogenicity, and safety of the HPV-16/18 AS04-adjuvanted vaccine: Final analysis of a long-term follow-up study up to 9.4 years post-vaccination. Human Vaccines & Immunotherapeutics. 2014;**10**(8):2147-2162. DOI: 10.4161/hv.29532

[111] Huh WK, Joura EA, Giuliano AR, Iversen OE, de Andrade RP, Ault KA, et al. Final efficacy, immunogenicity, and safety analyses of a nine-valent human papillomavirus vaccine in women aged 16-26 years: A randomised, double-blind trial. Lancet. 2017;**390**(10108):2143-2159. DOI: 10.1016/S0140-6736(17)31821-4

[112] Markowitz LE, Dunne EF, Saraiya M, Chesson HW, Curtis CR, Gee J, et al. Human papillomavirus vaccination: Recommendations of the Advisory Committee on Immunization Practices (ACIP). MMWR Recommendations and Reports. 2014;**63**(RR-05):1-30. Erratum in: MMWR Recommendations and Reports. 2014;**63**(49):1182

[113] Hildesheim A, Gonzalez P, Kreimer AR, Wacholder S, Schussler J, Rodriguez AC, et al. Impact of human papillomavirus (HPV) 16 and 18 vaccination on prevalent infections and rates of cervical lesions after excisional treatment. American Journal of Obstetrics & Gynecology. 2016;**215**(2):212.e1-212.e15. DOI: 10.1016/j.ajog.2016.02.021

[114] Hildesheim A, Herrero R, Wacholder S, Rodriguez AC, Solomon D, Bratti MC, et al. Effect of human papillomavirus 16/18 L1 viruslike particle vaccine among young women with preexisting infection: A randomized trial. Journal of the American Medical Association. 2007;**298**(7):743-753

[115] Hancock G, Hellner K, Dorrell L. Therapeutic HPV vaccines. Best Practice & Research Clinical Obstetrics & Gynaecology. 2018;**47**:59-72. DOI: 10.1016/j.bpobgyn.2017.09.008

[116] Trimble CL,Morrow MP, Kraynyak KA, Shen X, Dallas M, Yan J, et al. Safety, efficacy, and immunogenicity of VGX-3100, a therapeutic synthetic DNA vaccine targeting human papillomavirus 16 and 18 E6 and E7 proteins for cervical intraepithelial neoplasia 2/3: A randomised, double-blind, placebo-controlled phase 2b trial. Lancet. 2015;**386**(10008):2078-2088. DOI: 10.1016/S0140-6736(15)00239-1

[117] Yang A, Farmer E, Wu TC, Hung CF. Perspectives for therapeutic HPV vaccine development. Journal of Biomedical Science. 2016;**23**(1):75

[118] Faucette AN, Unger BL, Gonik B, Chen K. Maternal vaccination: Moving the science forward. Human Reproduction Update. 2015;**21**(1):119-135. DOI: 10.1093/humupd/dmu041

[119] Palmeira P, Quinello C, Silveira-Lessa AL, Zago CA, Carneiro-Sampaio M. IgG placental transfer in healthy and pathological pregnancies. Clinical & Developmental Immunology. 2012;**2012**:985646. DOI: 10.1155/2012/985646

[120] Chu HY, Englund JA. Maternal immunization. Birth Defects Research. 2017;**109**(5):379-386. DOI: 10.1002/bdra.23547

[121] Eberhardt CS, Blanchard-Rohner G, Lemaître B, Boukrid M, Combescure C, Othenin-Girard V, et al. Maternal immunization earlier in pregnancy maximizes antibody transfer and expected infant Seropositivity against pertussis. Clinical Infectious Diseases.

2016;**62**(7):829-836. DOI: 10.1093/cid/ciw027

[122] Eberhardt CS, Blanchard-Rohner G, Lemaître B, Combescure C, Othenin-Girard V, Chilin A, et al. Pertussis antibody transfer to preterm neonates after second- versus third-trimester maternal immunization. Clinical Infectious Diseases. 2017;**64**(8):1129-1132. DOI: 10.1093/cid/cix046

[123] Palmeira P, Carneiro-Sampaio M. Immunology of breast milk. Revista da Associação Médica Brasileira (1992). 2016;**62**(6):584-593. DOI: 10.1590/1806-9282.62.06.584

[124] De Schutter S, Maertens K, Baerts L, De Meester I, Van Damme P, Leuridan E. Quantification of vaccine-induced antipertussis toxin secretory IgA antibodies in breast milk: Comparison of different vaccination strategies in women. The Pediatric Infectious Disease Journal. 2015;**34**(6):e149-e152. DOI: 10.1097/INF.0000000000000675

[125] Niewiesk S. Maternal antibodies: Clinical significance, mechanism of interference with immune responses, and possible vaccination strategies. Frontiers in Immunology. 2014;**5**:446. DOI: 10.3389/fimmu.2014.00446

[126] Maertens K, Caboré RN, Huygen K, Vermeiren S, Hens N, Van Damme P, et al. Pertussis vaccination during pregnancy in Belgium: Follow-up of infants until 1 month after the fourth infant pertussis vaccination at 15 months of age. Vaccine. 2016;**34**(31):3613-3619. DOI: 10.1016/j.vaccine.2016.04.066

[127] Edwards KM. Maternal antibodies and infant immune responses to vaccines. Vaccine. 2015;**33**(47):6469-6472. DOI: 10.1016/j.vaccine.2015.07.085

[128] Amirthalingam G, Campbell H, Ribeiro S, Fry NK, Ramsay M, Miller E, et al. Sustained effectiveness of the maternal pertussis immunization program in England 3 years following introduction. Clinical Infectious Diseases. 2016;**63**(suppl 4):S236-S243

[129] Poland GA, Jacobson RM, Koutsky LA, Tamms GM, Railkar R, Smith JF, et al. Immunogenicity and reactogenicity of a novel vaccine for human papillomavirus 16: A 2-year randomized controlled clinical trial. Mayo Clinic Proceedings. 2005;**80**(5):601-610

[130] Human Papillomavirus Vaccines: WHO Position Paper, October 2014 [Internet]. Releve Epidemiologique Hebdomadaire. U.S. National Library of Medicine. 2014. Available from: https://www.ncbi.nlm.nih.gov/pubmed/25346960 [Cited Oct 10, 2019]

[131] Liu G, Kong L, Du P. HPV vaccine completion and dose adherence among commercially insured females aged 9 through 26 years in the US. Papillomavirus Research. 2016;**2**:1-8

[132] Bonde U, Joergensen JS, Lamont RF, Mogensen O. Is HPV vaccination in pregnancy safe? Human Vaccines & Immunotherapeutics. 2016;**12**(8):1960-1964. Epub May 12, 2016

Chapter 5

HPV Vaccines: Myths and Facts

Mehmet Faruk Kose and Emine Karabuk

Abstract

Many types of HPV virus found in nature are known to cause anogenital diseases and cancers in both of men and women. Genital condylomas caused by some types of HPV can cause important dermocosmetic, social, and psychological problems. On the other hand, cervical cancers caused by high-risk HPV types can be detected and treated in early stage or preinvasive period by using effective screening programs. But the main goal is to fight with the viruses causing the disease. Therefore, protective and preventive HPV virus vaccines are important. However, for effective administration of vaccines, it is necessary to know the effects of the vaccines, to whom it is applicable, any adverse effects, and to overcome prejudices against the vaccines and to clarify misinformation. In this chapter, in the light of current information about HPV vaccines, known facts and myths about vaccines are shared.

Keywords: HPV vaccines, cervical cancer, anogenital cancer, anogenital warts, efficacy, side effects

1. Introduction

The discovery of HPV (human papillomavirus) was awarded by Nobel Prize. Since 2008, when Prof. Dr. Harald zur Hausen (German Cancer Research Centre, Heidelberg, Germany) found the relationship between HPV and cervical cancer, the debate on HPV and its vaccine never ended (**Figure 1**).

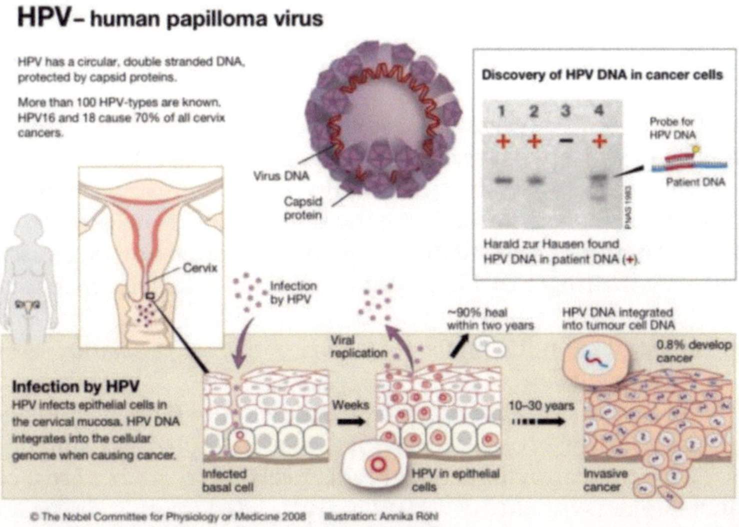

Figure 1.
HPV and cervical cancer (the Nobel Prize in Physiology or Medicine 2008).

There are more than 200 known types of HPV and 35–40 types are responsible for anogenital diseases. Fifteen high-risk types were also related to cancer. In order of their level of connection to cancer, the HPV types are: 16, 18, 45, 31, 33, 52, 58, 35, 59, 56, 51, 39, 68, 73, and 82. Out of those, 16 and 18 are responsible for 71–80% of the cancers and are five times more oncogenic than the other 13 types. From the low-risk types, 6 and 11 are responsible for 90% of the anogenital wart [1].

Looking geographically, 16, 18, 45, 31, 33, 52, and 58 are the seven most prevalent types, with little variation between locations [1]. In Turkey, Usubütün et al. found that types 16 and 18 had 76% prevalence in cervical cancers. The first six types (16, 18, 45, 31, 33, and 52) are responsible for 90.6% of the cancers [2].

In **Figure 2**, the full structure of both early (E) and late (L) proteins of HPV are shown, as well as their functions.

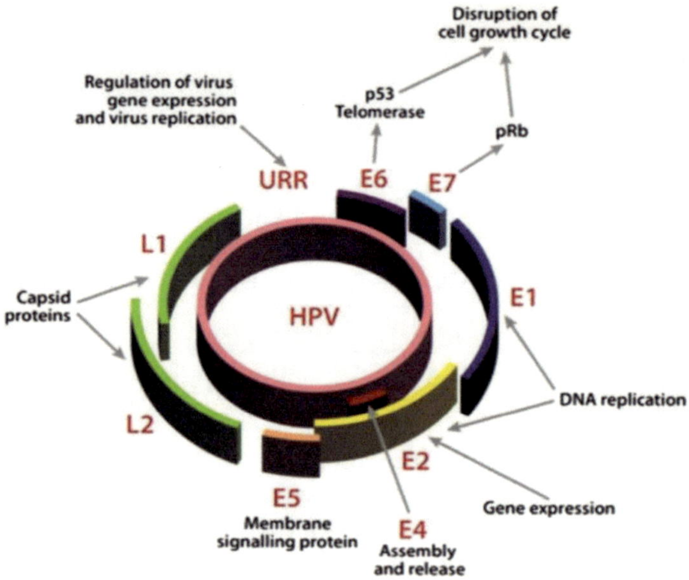

Figure 2.
L and E proteins of HPV and their functions.

In their lifetime, women have 80–85% chance to have an HPV infection, which means it is a widespread sexually transmitted disease. Speaking of sexually transmitted, 99% of all types are transmitted via sex, and using condoms do not protect from it (although some studies show that it protects up to 60%, theoretically any contact between testicals and the vulva is enough for transmission); it can spread even if a finger that had contact with the infected organ touches the opposite gender's genetelia (less than 0.1% of all cases), and since the virus requires body heat; it cannot be transmitted via pools, toilets, baths, saunas, or any other non-living surface.

So is HPV a cervical cancer factor, and are there other HPV-related diseases? HPV-related diseases are: cervix, anus, vulva, penis, oropharynx, and oral cavity cancers. The main reason for cervical cancer is HPV. In other words, cervical cancer cannot happen without HPV. HPV is also related to other diseases to some extent (**Figure 3**).

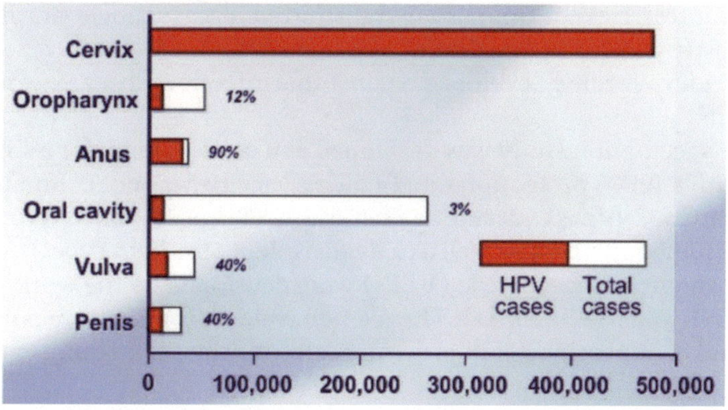

Figure 3.
HPV-related cancers and their HPV prevalence [3].

Recently, its association with lung cancer has been shown. In a study by Xiong et al. in 17 countries with 6890 cases and 7474 control groups, squamous cell carcinoma, adenocarcinoma and small-cell carcinoma types showed an increase post-HPV infection (Total OR 3.64 (95% CI: 2.60–5.08) for HPV 16: 3.14 (95% CI: 2.07–4.76) for HPV 18: 2.25 (95% CI: 1.49–3.40)) [4].

Apart from cancer, anogenital wart is one of the most important social problems. As seen in **Figure 4** for England and the Wales, anogenital wart increases with a country's level of development.

In Turkey, anogenital wart prevalence was found as 154/100,000 and in another study that was adjusted for age, point prevalence (lifetime incidence rate) was 3.8% for the full group, and 2.4% for the pregnant population. Prevalence study revealed similar results of recurrence with USA and Europe by 15–37% [5, 6].

The question, then, arises: Is HPV only for females? What about HPV in males? HPV has been shown to be associated with anogenital wart, anal and penile cancers in men [7, 8].

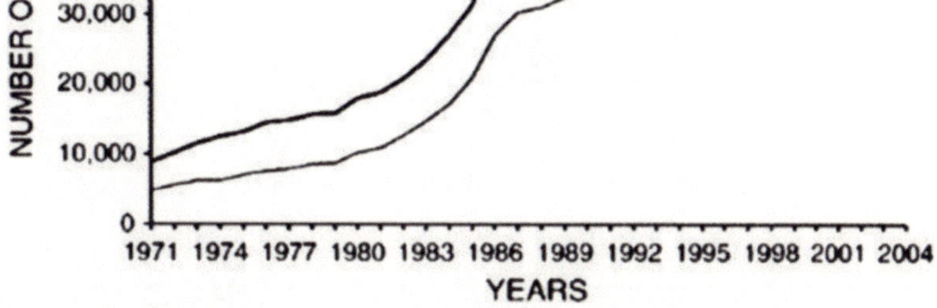

Figure 4.
Prevalence of anogenital wart in England and the Wales throughout the years (Health Protection Agency of England and Wales).

Males are the carriers of this sexual-transmitted disease; however, the disease burden is mostly present in females.

So, is there any vaccine developed against this infectious disease, can this disease be eliminated?

First ever vaccination study was developed as a monovalent (for a single type) against 16 with a 100% protection rate [9]. This vaccine was not commercialized.

A bivalent (for 2-types) vaccine against the most cancer-linked types 16 and 18 based on the previous study, as well as a quadrivalent (for four-types) vaccine based on recombinant virus-like particle (VLPs) were developed by the world-leader companies GSK and MSD [10, 11]. Then, a nonavalent (for nine-types) vaccine was developed and commercialized in order to protect against even more cancer-linked HPV types [12].

Since anogenital warts are one of the substantial social problems, it has not been available and bivalent vaccine against HPV 6 and 11 is still in progress. The current vaccines in use do not provide protection against HPV types associated with non-wart anogenital warts and non-melanoma skin cancers (NMSC). Therefore, vaccination studies against L2 proteins are in progress in the phase of animal experiments.

The International Papillomavirus Society, in an excerpt in the Guardian, pointed to Australia as a model for eradicating cervical cancer; they discussed results in between 2005 and 2015 and showed vaccination rates at 78.6% for girls below the age of 15 and 72.9% for boys below the age of 15, since 2016 [13].

World Health Organization (WHO) has developed a strategy plan to eliminate cervical cancer. According to the strategy, to provide a total elimination from cervical cancer, up to 15 years of age 90% of the girls should be vaccinated, 70% of females aged between 35 and 45 should be screened via high sensitivity tests and 90% of women should be successfully treated of cervical diseases (precancerous lesions and invasive cancers). World Health Organization stated that if these goals are reached by 2030, the elimination of cervical cancer would be possible in 2090 (**Figure 5**) (https://www.who.int/docs/defaultsource/documents/cervical-cancer-elimination-draft-strategy.pdf?sfvrsn=380979d6_4).

In Turkey, however, the situation is highly controversial. As of the last months of 2019, nonavalent is not licensed let alone being included in a vaccination programme. Unfortunately, two of our worst examples for vaccination; polio and hepatitis B; shows a 17-year delay in adapting vaccination programs behind the rest of the world. In 1955, there were statements on Milliyet Journal's columns such as

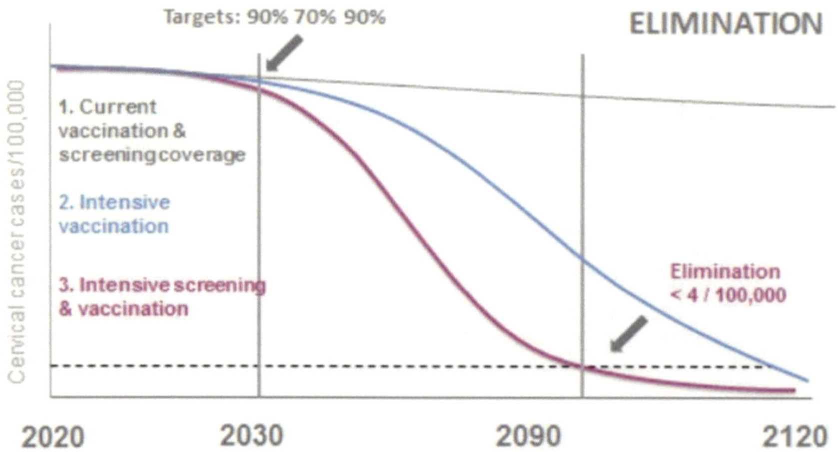

Figure 5.
Timeline for eliminating cervical cancer.

"The discovery of Polio vaccine caused a stir in Turkey" and "The news of Polio caused an excitement in our country but Turkish practitioners do not want to make any statement before getting informed from authorities." Seventeen years after these statements, polio was eliminated to be included in the vaccination programme of Turkey.

2. Myths

- Natural infection protects so there is no need for vaccination.
- Vaccinated children never experience HPV infection and never have HPV associated cancer throughout their lives.
- Vaccination cures their related disease.
- Antibody levels in blood are quite important; the protection loses its effect if the levels drop.
- Herd immunity (protection of the unvaccinated population) does not exist.
- Vaccinations are not effective when done at later ages.
- Smear or other HPV tests should be performed before the vaccination.
- If a pregnancy occurs during vaccination, it should be terminated.
- Vaccinated young girls have higher rates of sexually transmitted diseases since they feel more sexually comfortable.
- Autoimmune diseases such as primary ovarian deficiency and Guillain-Barre have higher rates among the vaccinated girls.
- There is cross-protection so vaccinations of HPV 16 and 18 are sufficient.
- If there is total protection against types in vaccinations, then cancer prevalence of other types will increase.
- Vaccines are not safe, there are deaths associated with the vaccine.
- Vaccines are not cost-effective, protected patients are not worth the cost.

3. Facts

3.1 Natural infection protects so there is no need for vaccination

HPV slithers through the cervical cracks and reaches basal cells in about 30 minutes and enters the cells to infect them. Since it does not stay in the vascular system, the antibody response does not form. Inside the cell, DNA is located episomally at first. Episomally located DNA causes a temporary infection and gets excreted with the cell when the cell is visible on the surface. If the DNA of the HPV gets integrated into the cell DNA, persistent infection will occur and some of them advance to preinvasive lesions. Only 15 of 100 HPV-infected women will develop cervical intraepithelial neoplasia (CIN) while 60% of them will have regression and 25% of them continue as infection.

In a study by Viscidi et al. with the National Cancer Institute (NCI) on the "Guanacaste, Costa Rica NCI Program," that included 10,049 women examined for over a 5-year period; natural HPV infection occurred on women independent of the type-based serological state. HPV infections from types 16, 18, and 31 rates were equal for both seronegative and seropositive cases. This is the clearest evidence which proves that natural infections do not protect against HPV [14].

3.2 Vaccinated children cannot get HPV or HPV-linked cancer in the future

Many patients as well as physicians have misinterpreted this issue. HPV-vaccinated patients that develop HPV-related diseases are shown as exemplary cases. What is the right information, then? Considering the cervical cancer, only 15 high-risk types can cause cancer. Types 16 and 18 that are included in the vaccines are responsible for 71–76% and the seven high-risk types in the nonavalent vaccines are responsible for 88–90% of all cervical cancer. Naturally, even nonavalent vaccines do not protect against all HPV types, and HPV infection can develop in the rest. Furthermore, we know that LSIL (low-grade squamous intraepithelial lesion) may develop not only through high-risk HPV types but also it can be caused by other types of HPV.

In the end, naïve (no prior contact with HPV) group children are protected close to 100% against *the types included in the vaccine*. Adults who have not developed the same type HPV before are also protected close to 100%. If they developed it before, they are instead protected against the other included types.

However, FUTURE III study shows us that the chance of developing both types 16 and 18 infections is less than 1% [15]. In addition to this, Kang et al. studied the efficacy of quadrivalent vaccines in 737 cases treated for CIN 3 over the course of 3 years. In this randomized controlled study, 360 vaccinated cases and 377 non-vaccinated cases were monitored in terms of recurrent diseases associated with certain HPV types. In the vaccinated group, recurrent infection rate was 2.5% while in the non-vaccinated group, the rate was 8.5% (HR = 2.840; CI: 1.335–6.042; $p < 0.01$) [16].

As a summary, both vaccinated girls and boys can develop HPV infections, which can lead to cancer, with types that are not included in the vaccine. Anogenital warts can occur with HPV types other than 6 and 11, hence the quadrivalent and nonavalent vaccinated group can develop anogenital warts at a rate lower than 10%.

3.3 Vaccination cures their related disease

Vaccines do not treat HPV-associated diseases. They are not therapeutic. However, as stated in previous section, vaccines are effective in preventing recurrent infections.

3.4 Antibody levels in blood are quite important; the protection loses its effect if the levels drop

Both bivalent and quadrivalent HPV vaccines' fundamental studies, FUTURE [15] and PATRICIA [17], recorded related blood antibody levels. In these studies, neutralizing antibody levels were measured for four different age groups: 15–25, 26–35, 36–45, and 46–55 years old. For per protocol groups, both HPV 16 and 18 neutralizing antibodies separately showed a peak at 7 months (after the third dose).

Antibody levels were found to be at least 8 times higher compared to natural infections, even in the youngest age group. HPV vaccines were found to have a general characteristic to be effective when done in both childhood and later ages. Neutralizing antibody level of 4V HPV vaccine for type 18 started to fall starting at 24 months and fell to the natural infection level at 55 months. Neutralizing antibodies showed 76% decrease at 24 weeks and 56% at 36 weeks.

Does this decrease in antibody level correspond to a decrease in protection level against type 18? In a 2008 RCT study by Joura et al., the protection level against HPV type 18 was steady at 98.4% (95% CI: 90.5–100) even when the antibody levels fell [18]. Ault et al. also showed that at 4 years mark, CIN 2/3 protection levels were at 100% even when seropositivity dropped to 60% [19]. When we consider the HPV vaccinated population that did not follow the full protocol; or had one or two doses only, by the 15th year mark hepatitis B vaccine shows a similar result. One or two dose vaccination was shown to provide comparable protection to three-dose regimes [20]. Even though hepatitis B vaccinated population's neutralizing antibody level was not measurable, the protection level was known to be still at 100%. This goal is presumed to be reflected on HPV vaccination soon. As in, changes in the neutralizing antibody levels do not affect the protection, which will stay at 100%.

3.5 Herd immunity does not exist

Herd immunity, or the increase in protection rate of the unvaccinated population as the overall vaccination rate increases, is a well-known fact for all types of vaccines. In Sweden, even though quadrivalent HPV vaccination rates are very low, 15–44 years old unvaccinated men and women had significant decrease on the annual rate-of-change percentage [21]. Therefore, as the community vaccination rate increases, those who are not vaccinated with HPV-related vaccines will develop HPV-related diseases at a lower rate.

3.6 Vaccinations are not effective when done at later ages

It was shown that HPV vaccination generates high neutralizing antibody levels when done in early childhood as well as at later ages. PATRICIA and FUTURE studies, at four age groups of 15–25, 26–35, 36–45 and 46–55 years old, shows consistent antibody levels for all of them. Even if there is not a statistical significance on vaccination of the naïve population, it is expected to be more effective. However, for all three vaccinations, EMA (European Medicine Agency) does not provide a set age limit. After considering the available data and studies, EMA decided to lift the age limit on women. However, there is a soft 25 years-old upper limit for men. This age limit is due to follow-up case series not being available yet.

3.7 Smear or other HPV tests should be performed before the vaccination

Vaccination will not protect against infections that occurred prior to it. FUTURE III study shows us that developing both HPV 16 and 18 together has a chance less than 1%. According to abnormal smear results, HSIL and cancer are only correlated with high-risk HPV types. On the other hand, LSIL is correlated with both high-risk HPV types as well as others. Hence, HPV DNA test prior to vaccination can only tell for less than 1% of women if the vaccine cannot protect against the most prevalent types 16 and 18. Studies also show that vaccinations help reduce reinfection rate for prior type 16 and/or 18 infections. On top of the infections, a randomized control study on LEEP treated cases due to HSIL, shows us that vaccinated group had a reduced reinfection rate at 2.5% compared to 8.5% [16]. According to this data, smear or HPV DNA tests are not required prior to vaccination.

3.8 If a pregnancy occurs during vaccination, it should be terminated

There are limited number of cases about uses of bivalent and quadrivalent HPV vaccination during pregnancy. Both vaccines are classified as category B due to prior data. Comparison between vaccinated and unvaccinated group did not show an increase in the infant's congenital anomaly rates. However, due to unavailability of more data, vaccination during pregnancy is not recommended. This does not mean that the vaccination is done without knowledge of the pregnancy, that it should be aborted [22].

3.9 Due to decreased sexual fear, sexually transmitted disease rates increase among vaccinated girls

From a social, psychologic, and religious angle; parents of vaccinated girls wonder if the protection of the vaccine would urge them to be more sexually active at a younger age. It would be an issue if it was true. In order to answer this, a study published at Pediatrics reported sexually transmitted infections (STI) history of vaccinated girls. Mayhew et al. found that between the 42.5% cases without prior sexual relations and 57.5% cases with prior sexual relations, there was only a difference of OR 0:13 (95% CI: 0.03–0.69) which shows that vaccination did not change their sexual behavior [23].

3.10 Autoimmune diseases such as primary ovarian insufficiency and Guillain-Barre have higher rates among the vaccinated girls

In order to claim that a vaccination developed a disease, it needs to be within 3 years. At the 9th-year mark of HPV vaccines, 170,000,000 doses of vaccines had been done. Out of this large sample size, only six cases in the literature show primer ovarian insufficiency. Looking closer, we see that three of these cases had irregular periods up to 15 years before vaccination. The other three cases had their diagnosis more than 3 years after vaccination [24].

In the placebo-controlled FUTURE III (quadrivalent HPV vaccine) study, in both the vaccinated and AAHS (regular saline, placebo) groups, autoimmune disease rates were at 2.3%. This is the clearest study that shows autoimmune disease rate does not increase in vaccinated population. In addition, in a large meta-analysis study by Genovese et al. (243,289 vaccinated and 248,820 control group) there was no correlation between HPV vaccines and autoimmune diseases [25].

3.11 Vaccines that include types 16 and 18 are enough for the rest due to cross-protection effect

The difference between cross-protection and cross-reaction is an important issue. Bivalent and quadrivalent HPV vaccines both show cross-reaction. Especially in bivalent HPV vaccines, researchers argued for cross-protection due to common ancestry of types 16 and 31 as well as 18 and 45. In bivalent vaccinated girls, HPV 31 and 45 immune response, as well as GMTs and seropositivity rates were considered. Serum GMTs were 20 times higher than natural infections for HPV 31 and 45. This effect, however, is cross-reaction. Because the vaccinated girls and women lose the protection against HPV 31 and 45 by the end of 4th year in these bivalent HPV studies [26–28].

In a report by the Centers for Disease Control and Prevention (CDC) in the USA, as of 2018, there are no bivalent or quadrivalent HPV vaccines in the market; only nonavalent HPV vaccine is sold [29].

3.12 If the vaccines include full protection against some types, cancer rates in the rest of the types will increase

This is a baseless theory from anti-vaccination group. Is it necessary to prove the opposite of this theory? Even so, there have been studies on the matter. In 1180 vaccinated cases, anogenital non-vaccinated type HPV and genetic-related HPV 16 and 18 types prevalence are studied. There was no change in the non-vaccinated HPV type prevalence [30].

3.13 Vaccines are not safe; there are deaths associated with the vaccine

Three independent institutes on the CDC Website are continuously monitoring the safety of vaccines and the data is available for both experts and the community. Because in the USA, every drug that is on the market has an obligation for routine control. These vaccine-monitoring systems are: the Vaccine Adverse Event Reporting System (VAERS), the Vaccine Safety Datalink (VSD), and the Clinical Immunization Safety Assessment (CISA) Network; and any person who had an adverse effect from a vaccine can report to them freely.

Vaccines consist of VLPs (virus-like particles) made with recombinant technology, that do not include any DNA but are identical to HPV in terms of structure. They cannot develop HPV infections or HPV-related cancer, as they do not include any DNA to reproduce. On the other hand, weakened or killed bacteria or virus vaccines do have a minute risk [31].

Side effects include redness in the vaccination site, minor pain, inflammation, and mild fever; like all childhood vaccinations. It could also cause nausea and dizziness. Due to this, vaccinated people are recommended to rest for 15 minutes after. VAERS records show that when divided into critical side effects and non-critical side effects; side effect rates were on a steady decline since 2007. In theory, autoimmune diseases are the most common side effect claims. In a quadrivalent HPV vaccine in 1000 cases of 9–26 year-old girls and women, there were no differences in autoimmune diseases between the vaccine group and the adjuvant or physiologic serum group. Both groups reported a rate of 2.3%.

When nonavalent HPV vaccine was introduced after the quadrivalent vaccine, which had twice the amount of aluminum (500 μg = 0.5 mg) of the latter, several anti-vaccination physicians theorized that this would worsen the side effects. However, any side effect of the 0.5 mg AAHS in hepatitis B, which has been used for 25 years, has never been proven. In a new study on the safety of aluminum in vaccines, the aluminum in the immunity-booster adjuvants had a high safety factor and did not cause any neurotoxicity [32]. Furthermore, we ingest more aluminum from drinking water (<0.2 ml/L), from many foods such as potatoes and spinach (<5 mg/kg), from aluminum folio to preserve food, from food with aluminum supplements, and soy-based food (0.4–6 mg/L) compared to the vaccines (https://www.cfs.gov.hk/.../files/RA35_Aluminium_in_Food_e.pdf).

Theory that quadrivalent and nonavalent HPV vaccines can cause primary ovarian insufficiency (POI) has been claimed by experts in many places including the social media. As described in detail in the previous section, there have been only 6 POI cases out of 170,000,000 doses of HPV vaccines in over 9 years. What is the incidence rate of POI in a normal population? Spontaneous POI for under

30-years old is about 0.1%, and for under 40-years old is about 1%. In Australia, out of 5,800,000 doses for 83% school-age girls, there was no relation between HPV and POI [33].

In Japan, there is a two-staged national vaccine program; quadrivalent HPV vaccine was implemented to the first stage in 2010 and was moved to the second stage in April 2013. This allowed only anyone that wanted to be vaccinated. The reason was abnormal uterus bleeding, excessive uterus bleeding, and headache. To address this, 71,117 women were studied and no relation between the symptoms and vaccination were found. As a result, vaccines were reimplemented into the first stage in June 2013 [34].

Considering mortality, CDC Website reports 117 deaths for the 80,000,000 doses of vaccines from the related institutes and 51 of them had a known cause. These known causes were unrelated to vaccines. Recorded death causes included: traffic accident, homicide, epilepsy crisis for epilepsy diagnosed patients, pulmonary embolism, drug overdose for drug abuse patients, acute myocarditis, and meningoencephalitis, influenza B, and diabetic ketoacidosis. There were five reported deaths after nonavalent vaccines were introduced: car accident, suicide, acute lymphoblastic leukemia, septic shock, and an unknown cause. There are many meta-analysis and reviews about vaccine safety readily available. There are no differences in between vaccinated and unvaccinated groups in terms of critical side effects.

3.14 Vaccines are not cost-effective; protected patients are not worth the cost

This is an interesting claim. Every single patient protected is worth the effort. Looking through a scientific perspective, many studies found that even the vaccines based on HPV 6/11 related warts, HPV 16/18 related precancerous lesions, and cervical cancer are cost effective [35–37].

4. Conclusion

HPV vaccines are recommended by WHO, CDC that are the world's leading organizations, and related associations of all other developed countries, have not yet reached the deserved coverage rate. WHO described HPV vaccination as an essential part of its program when talking about the elimination of cervical cancer. The most well-known topic of all medical staff is "The worst vaccine is better than the best treatment." As such, there are numbers of myths about HPV vaccines that we mentioned above. These issues should be well known to all of our community, especially health professionals, so that HPV vaccination can become widespread. We wanted to share the truths of these myths with you in the light of the evidences of today. In this article, neither of us have any conflict of interest.

DOI: http://dx.doi.org/10.5772/intechopen.90442

Author details

Mehmet Faruk Kose[1*] and Emine Karabuk[2]

1 Department of Gynecologic and Oncology, School of Medicine, Acibadem Mehmet Ali Aydinlar University, Turkey

2 Department of Obstetrics and Gynecology, School of Medicine, Acibadem Mehmet Ali Aydinlar University, Turkey

*Address all correspondence to: mfarukkose@gmail.com

References

[1] Munoz N, Bosch FX, Castellsague X, Díaz M, de Sanjose S, Hammouda D, et al. Against which human papillomavirus types shall we vaccinate and screen? The international perspective. International Journal of Cancer. 2004;**111**(2):278-285

[2] Usubütün A, Alemany L, Kucukali T, Ayhan A, et al. Human papillomavirus types in invasive cervical cancer specimens from Turkey. International Journal of Gynecological Pathology. 2009;**28**(6):541-548

[3] Parkin DM, Bray F. The burden of HPV-related cancers. Vaccine. 2006;**24**(Suppl 3):S3/11-S3/25

[4] Xiong WM, Xu QP, Li X, Xiao RD, Cai L, He F. The association between human papilloma-virus infection and lung cancer: A system review and meta-analysis. Oncotarget. 2017;**8**(56):96419-96432

[5] Ozgul N, Tuncer M, Abacioglu M, Gultekin M. Estimating prevalence of genital warts in Turkey: Survey among KETEM-affiliated gynecologists across Turkey. Asian Pacific Journal of Cancer Prevention. 2011;**12**(9):2397-2400

[6] Kose MF, Akin L, Yuce K, Turkish Society for Colposcopy, Cervical Pathology Study Group. Prevalence of genital warts in reproductive-aged Turkish women presenting at gynecology outpatient clinics for any reason. Clinical and Experimental Obstetrics & Gynecology. 2013;**40**(3):407-414

[7] Daling JR, Madeleine MM, Johnson LG, Schwartz SM, et al. Penile cancer: Importance of circumcision, human papillomavirus and smoking in in situ and invasive disease. International Journal of Cancer. 2005;**116**(4):606-616

[8] Daling JR, Madeleine MM, Johnson LG, Schwartz SM, et al. Human papillomavirus, smoking, and sexual practices in the etiology of anal cancer. Cancer. 2004;**101**(2):270-280

[9] Rowhani-Rahbar A, Mao C, Hughes JP, Alvarez FB, et al. Longer term efficacy of a prophylactic monovalent human papillomavirus type 16 vaccine. Vaccine. 2009;**27**(41):5612-5619

[10] Paavonen J, Jenkins D, Bosch FX, Naud P, Salmerón J, et al. Efficacy of a prophylactic adjuvanted bivalent L1 virus-like-particle vaccine against infection with human papillomavirus types 16 and 18 in young women: An interim analysis of a phase III double-blind, randomised controlled trial. Lancet. 2007;**369**(9580):2161-2170

[11] FUTURE II Study Group. Quadrivalent vaccine against human papillomavirus to prevent high grade cervical lesions. The New England Journal of Medicine. 2007;**356**(19):1915-1927

[12] Chatterjee A. The next generation of HPV vaccines: Nonavalent vaccine V503 on the horizon. Expert Review of Vaccines. 2014;**13**(11):1279-1290

[13] Korostil IA, Ali H, Guy RJ, Donovan B, Law MG, Regan DG. Near elimination of genital warts in Australia predicted with extension of human papillomavirus vaccination to males. Sexually Transmitted Diseases. 2013;**40**(11):833-835

[14] Viscidi RP, Schiffman M, Hildesheim A, Herrero R, Castle PE, Bratti MC, et al. Seroreactivity to human papillomavirus (HPV) types 16, 18, or 31 and risk of subsequent HPV infection: Results from a population-based study in Costa Rica.

Cancer Epidemiology, Biomarkers & Prevention. 2004;**13**(2):324-327

[15] Munoz N, Manalastas R Jr, Pitisuttithum P, Tresukosol D, et al. Safety, immunogenicity, and efficacy of quadrivalent human papillomavirus (types 6, 11, 16, 18) recombinant vaccine in women aged 24-45 years: A randomised, double-blind trial. Lancet. 2009;**373**(9679):1949-1957

[16] Kang WD, Choi HS, Kim SM. Is vaccination with quadrivalent HPV vaccine after loop electrosurgical excision procedure effective in preventing recurrence in patients with high grade cervical intraepithelial neoplasia (CIN2-3)? Gynecologic Oncology. 2013;**130**(2):264-268

[17] Kreimer AR, Struyf F, Del Rosario-Raymundo MR, Hildesheim A, Skinner SR, Wacholder S, et al. Efficacy of fewer than three doses of an HPV-16/18 AS04-adjuvanted vaccine: Combined analysis of data from the Costa Rica Vaccine and PATRICIA Trials. The Lancet Oncology. 2015;**16**(7):775-786

[18] Joura EA, Kjaer SK, Wheeler CM, Sigurdsson K, Iversen OE, Hernandez-Avila M, et al. HPV antibody levels and clinical efficacy following administration of a prophylactic quadrivalent HPV vaccine. Vaccine. 2008;**26**(52):6844-6851

[19] Ault K, for the FUTURE I and II Study Group (FR). Impact of quadrivalent HPV (Type 6, 11, 16, 18) vaccine on HPV 18-related disease including adenocarcinoma of the cervix. In: 20th European Congress of Obstetrics and Gynaecology. 2008

[20] Kjaer SK, Sigurdsson K, Iversen OE, Hernandez-Avila M, Wheeler CM, Perez G, et al. A pooled analysis of continued prophylactic efficacy of quadrivalent human papillomavirus (types 6/11/16/18) vaccine against high-grade cervical and external genital lesions. Cancer Prevention Research (Philadelphia, Pa.). 2009;**2**(10):868-878

[21] Sampson JN, Hildesheim A, Herrero R, Gonzalez P, Kreimer AR, Gail MH. Design and statistical considerations for studies evaluating the efficacy of a single dose of the human papillomavirus (HPV) vaccine. Contemporary Clinical Trials. 2018;**68**:35-44. DOI: 10.1016/j.cct.2018.02.010

[22] Herweijer E, Ploner A, Sparén P. Substantially reduced incidence of genital warts in women and men six years after HPV vaccine availability in Sweden. Vaccine. 2018;**36**(15):1917-1920

[23] Descamps D, Hardt K, Spiessens B, Izurieta P, Verstraeten T, Breuer T, et al. Safety of human papillomavirus (HPV)-16/18 AS04-adjuvanted vaccine for cervical cancer prevention: A pooled analysis of 11 clinical trials. Human Vaccines. 2009;**5**(5):332-340

[24] Mayhew A, Mullins TL, Ding L, Rosenthal SL, Zimet GD, Morrow C, et al. Risk perceptions and subsequent sexual behaviors after HPV vaccination in adolescents. Pediatrics. 2014;**133**(3):404-411

[25] Little DT, Ward HR. Adolescent premature ovarian insufficiency following human papillomavirus vaccination: A case series seen in general practice. Journal of Investigative Medicine High Impact Case Reports. Oct-Dec 2014;**2**(4):1-12

[26] Genovese C, LA Fauci V, Squeri A, Trimarchi G, Squeri R. HPV vaccine and autoimmune diseases: Systematic review and meta-analysis of the literature. Journal of Preventive Medicine and Hygiene. 2018;**59**(3):E194-E199

[27] Romanowski B. Long term protection against cervical infection with the human papillomavirus: Review of currently available vaccines. Human Vaccines. 2011;**7**(2):161-169

[28] Safaeian M, Kemp TJ, Pan DY, Porras C, Rodriguez AC, Schiffman M, et al. Cross-protective vaccine efficacy of the bivalent HPV vaccine against HPV31 is associated with humoral immune responses: Results from the Costa Rica Vaccine Trial. Human Vaccines & Immunotherapeutics. 2013;**9**(7):1399-1406

[29] Dilley S, Miller K, Huh W. HPV vaccination. Gynecologic Oncology. 2018;**148**(1):3-4

[30] Saccucci M, Franco EL, Ding L, Bernstein DI, Brown D, Kahn JA. Non-vaccine-type human papillomavirus prevalence after vaccine introduction: No evidence for type replacement but evidence for cross-protection. Sexually Transmitted Diseases. 2018;**45**(4):260-265

[31] Kirnbauer R, Booy F, Cheng N, Lowy DR, Schiller JT. Papillomavirus L1 major capsid protein self-assembles into virus-like particles that are highly immunogenic. Proceedings of the National Academy of Sciences of the United States of America. 1992;**89**(24):12180-12184

[32] Principi N, Esposito S. Aluminum in vaccines: Does it create a safety problem? Vaccine. 2018;**36**(39):5825-5831

[33] Little DT, Ward HR. Ongoing inadequacy of quadrivalent HPV vaccine safety studies. BMJ Evidence-Based Medicine. 7 Jan 2019; pii: bmjebm-2018-111122

[34] Suzuki S, Hosono A. No association between HPV vaccine and reported post-vaccination symptoms in Japanese young women: Results of the Nagoya study. Papillomavirus Research. 2018;**5**:96-103

[35] Connelly LB, Le HN. Cost-effectiveness of a bivalent human papillomavirus vaccination program in Japan. Sexual Health. 2015;**12**(6):520-531

[36] Annemans L, Rémy V, Oyee J, Largeron N. Cost-effectiveness evaluation of a quadrivalent human papillomavirus vaccine in Belgium. PharmacoEconomics. 2009;**27**(3):231-245

[37] Armstrong EP. Prophylaxis of cervical cancer and related cervical disease: A review of the cost-effectiveness of vaccination against oncogenic HPV types. Journal of Managed Care Pharmacy. 2010;**16**(3):217-230

Chapter 6

HPV and Cervical Cancer Control Programs: Effective Translation of Knowledge into Practice

Rajamanickam Rajkumar

Abstract

Cervical cancer is a major cancer affecting 5.3 million women annually, worldwide, and is responsible for about 2.7 million deaths per year. More than 85% of the incident cases occur in developing countries. Cervical cancer is a totally preventable cancer, if diagnosed in the precancer stages and treated effectively. HPV vaccination has been introduced in many countries. Effective screening and treatment programs are available in many health settings. Posttreatment histopathological follow-up is done for 3–5 years. Cure from precancer condition and prevention of invasive cervical cancer are thus attained. But the main hurdle in achieving the above ambitious goal is the lacunae and deficiencies in conversion of knowledge into practice by the women who are otherwise well informed about the prevention of cervical cancer, as result of massive inputs in the field of health education. Thus, the screening participation and compliance to precancer treatment remain low. This barrier in translational knowledge should be overcome efficiently. **The author, from his vast experience in planning and implementing one of the largest cervical cancer screening programs in India, has conceptualized** "the STAR model P6 principles of Raj" for successful conversion of "knowledge into practice."

Keywords: cervical cancer, screening, treatment, low participation, translational knowledge to practice

1. Introduction

Cervical cancer is the fourth common cancer among women in the world, and it accounts for about 530,000 new cases and 270,000 deaths annually, as reported in 2012. About 85% of these cases occur in developing countries. It represents 12% of incident cancers in women and 7.5% deaths due to cancer in women.

In a developing country like India, about 122,000 new cases of cervical cancer and about 67,400 deaths due cervical cancer are reported, every year, as per data of 2017. It is the second most frequent cancer among women of reproductive age group.

India also has the highest age standardized incidence of cervical cancer in South Asia at 22, compared to 19.2 in Bangladesh, 13 in Sri Lanka, and 2.8 in Iran [1, 2].

2. The role of HPV

HPV is a necessary cause for cervical cancer [3].

More than 115 types of HPV are present and 18 are high-risk carcinogenic types for cervical cancer. Other than this, HPV-16 is the most common high risk in cervical cancer [4].

In cervical cancer cases, HPV prevalence was in the range of 87.8 to 96.67%, in a study in India. In women without cervical cancer, HPV prevalence varied from 7.5 to 16.9%.

The worldwide prevalence of HPV infection, in normal woman, is between 9% and 13%.

3. HPV infection worldwide

HPV is associated with 50,000 new cases of cervical cancer and 250,000 associated cervical cancer deaths, worldwide, each year [5]. It also causes vulvar, vaginal, anal, and penile cancers and precancerous lesions of vulva/vagina, genital warts, and respiratory papilomatosis [5–7]. HPV infections are asymptomatic, and generally, individuals are not aware of being infected, thus facilitating the spread easily and unknowingly [5].

At least 50% of men and women will acquire genital HPV infection during their lifetime [8].

All sexually active women are infected with HPV at least once during their lifetime, and the highest prevalence is seen soon after the onset of sexual activities [9, 10].

A majority of episodes of type-specific HPV infection resolve spontaneously within 2 years, but this may be followed by an infection with a new type [7].

HPV transmission exclusively occurs following skin-to-skin contact with an infected partner. Sexual intercourse is not necessary, and the virus can be transmitted through sexual foreplay [5].

HPV can only replicate in the stratified squamous epithelium. HPV infection is the most common sexually transmitted diseases [11]. The major risk factor for HPV infection is sexual behavior, including early age of onset of sexual activity, multiple sexual partners, and coinfection with HIV [12].

Although the determinants of risk for persistent infection and progression to invasive diseases are not fully understood, persistence appears to be related to HPV type and concurrent infection with multiple virus types [12].

The prevalence and distribution of HPV types in the general population as well as in cervical neoplasia vary with geographic region and by the grade of disease [13].

4. Screening for cervical cancer

Secondary prevention involves screening for precancerous lesions and treating them. The three screening modalities are cytology, visual inspection, and HPV test.

5. Prevention of cervical cancer

HPV is necessary for the development of cervical cancer. Therefore, preventing HPV infection can prevent cervical cancer. This can be achieved by complete abstinence from sexual activity or by a vaccine [14].

Primary prevention involves a risk reduction approach through behavioral intervention for sexual and healthcare-seeking behavior or through mass immunization against high-risk HPV [15].

The objective of cervical screening/secondary prevention is to prevent invasive cervical cancer from developing by detecting and treating women with CIN2/3 lesions, and the effectiveness is determined by reduction in incidence and mortality.

The critical components of a screening program are an acceptable good-quality screening test, prompt diagnostic investigations, appropriate treatment, and posttreatment follow-up [16].

There is a strong support from nonexperimental studies in developed countries such as Denmark and Finland that the incidence and mortality of cervical cancer can be reduced by screening [17].

Ensuring high levels of participation and sufficient healthcare infrastructure and human resources are important for a screening program to succeed [18]. It is also important for screening to be guided by equity considerations for those who are more vulnerable or with lesser access to healthcare services because of social, economic, or demographic factors [19].

Recent screening recommendations for specific age groups as per the American Cancer Society (ACS) screening guidelines are as follows: [1, 2].

- At the age of 21 years: Screening is recommended.
- At the age of 21–29 years: Cytology (Pap smear) alone every 3 years.
- At the age of 30–65 years: Human papillomavirus virus (HPV) and cytology contesting every 5 years or cytology alone every 3 years.
- At the age of >65 years: No screening recommended if adequate prior screening has been negative and high risk is not present.

HPV Vaccines that aims to prevent cervical cancer are:

- A bivalent vaccine which protects against subtypes 16 and 18.
- A quadrivalent vaccine which protects against subtypes 16 and 18 plus 6 and 11.
- A 9-valent vaccine which protects against the same subtypes as the quadrivalent plus subtypes 31, 33, 45, 52, and 58 (which cause about 15% of cervical cancers).
- The HPV vaccine is ideally recommended to vaccinate boys and girls at age 11–12 years, but vaccination can begins at age 9.

6. The effect of HPV vaccination

1. Population-level impact and herd effects following the introduction of human papillomavirus vaccination programs

From the abstract: We did a systematic review and meta-analysis of the population-level impact of vaccinating girls and women against human papillomavirus on HPV infections, anogenital wart diagnoses, and cervical intraepithelial neoplasia grade 2+ (CIN2+). Our results show compelling evidence of the substantial impact of HPV vaccination programs on HPV infections and CIN2+ among girls and women, and on anogenital warts diagnoses among girls, women, boys, and men, programs with multi-cohort vaccination and high vaccination coverage had a greater direct impact and herd effects.

Ref: *Population-level impact and herd effects following the introduction of human papillomavirus vaccination programmes: updated systematic review and meta-analysis*

Drolet M, Bénard É, Pérez N, Brisson M, on behalf of the HPV Vaccination Impact Study Group. The Lancet. Open access

2. Human papillomavirus (HPV) vaccination significantly reduces the frequency of genital HPV 16 and 18 infections and cervical intraepithelial neoplasia grade 2+ (CIN2+) in young women and shows signs of herd effects with a reduced frequency of anogenital warts in both young women and men, a recent study showed.

As cited in infectious diseases.

9/16/2019 HPV vaccination programmes reduce HPV infection, precancerous lesions with potential crossover and herd effects | News for Doctor, N.

https://specialty.mims.com/topic/hpv-vaccination-programmes-reduce-hpv-infection–precancerous-lesions-with-potential-crossover-and-herd-effects-? ... 1/7.

7. KAP studies reveal the presence of adequate knowledge but inadequate "practice "in the community

7.1 Recent study in India

Results: We observed that despite good knowledge and perception, less than 10 percent of workers have undergone screening. Significant association was seen between the level of knowledge and practice of screening.

Conclusion: It is of utmost importance narrowing of existing gap between the perception and practice of cervical cancer.

Screening should be initiated through introducing more educational programs for workers and encouraging them to participate.

The study cited is from: Khanna D, Khargekar N, Budukh A. Knowledge, attitude, and practice about cervical cancer and its screening among community healthcare workers of Varanasi district, Uttar Pradesh, India. J Family Med Prim Care 2019;8:1715–9.

8. How to translate "knowledge" in to "practice"

Author's experiences in a cervical cancer screening program of the IARC/WHO, In India.

8.1 The development of the STAR model P-6 principles of raj©

The author, having been successful in planning and implementing, such a model, and achieving a reduction in the incidence rate of cervical cancer by 25% and mortality due to cervical cancer by 35%, in a period of 7 years—2000 to 2007, strongly recommends the STAR model P-6 principles of Raj©.

He has served as the principal investigator for the first 3 years, and the project was done at the Christian Fellowship Community Health Centre Society, Ambilikkai, Dindigul district, Tamil Nadu, India, and was in technical collaboration with the International Agency for Research on Cancer (IARC), WHO.

9. Background

Proof of concept (POC)—The Lancet Publication 2007, the author's paper.

Quote:

Effect of visual screening on cervical cancer incidence and mortality in Tamil Nadu, India: a cluster-randomized trial.

Lancet 2007; 370(9585):398-406.

Rengaswamy Sankaranarayanan, Pulikkottil Okkuru Esmy, Rajamanickam Rajkumar, et al.

10. Summary

Cervical cancer is the most common cancer among women in developing countries. We assessed the effect of screening using visual inspection with 4% acetic acid (VIA) on cervical cancer incidence and mortality in a cluster-randomized controlled trial in India.

11. Methods

Of the 114 study clusters in Dindigul district, India, 57 were randomized to one round of VIA by trained nurses and 57 to a control group. Healthy women aged 30–59 years were eligible for the study. Screen-positive women had colposcopy, directed biopsies, and, where appropriate, cryotherapy by nurses during the screening visit. Those with larger precancerous lesions or invasive cancers were referred for appropriate investigations and treatment.

Cervical cancer incidence and mortality in the study groups were analyzed and compared using Cox regression taking the cluster design into account, and analysis was by intention to treat. The primary outcome measures were cervical cancer incidence and mortality.

12. Results

Of the 49,311 eligible women in the intervention group, 31,343 (63·6%) were screened during 2000–2003; 30,958 control women received the standard care. Of the 3088 (9·9%) screened positive, 3052 had colposcopy and 2539 directed biopsy. Of the 1874 women with precancerous lesions in the intervention group, 72% received treatment. In the intervention group, 274,430 person years, 167 cervical cancer cases, and 83 cervical cancer deaths were accrued compared with 178,781 person years, 158 cases, and 92 deaths and in the control group during 2000–2006 (incidence hazard ratio 0·75 [95% CI 0·55–0·95] and mortality hazard ratio 0·65 [0·47–0·89]).

13. Interpretation

HPV vaccination and organized screening, in the presence of good training and sustained quality assurance, are effective methods, for HPV and cervical cancer prevention and control, in developing countries. New and innovative models and effective strategies for health education need to be developed to strengthen the "knowledge translation to action" component of the healthcare delivery systems,

14. Health education: for HPV prevention and control

The STAR model P-6 principles of Raj©.

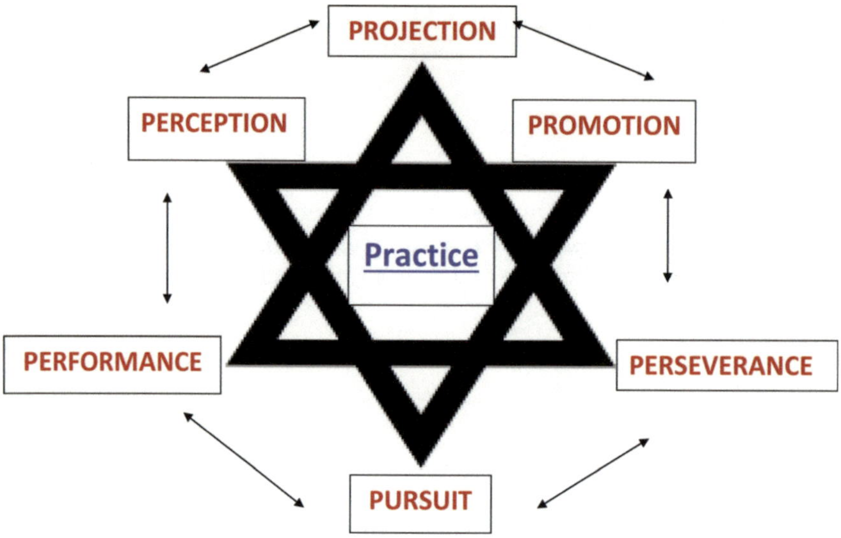

Health education, with special strategies to effect the "practice" in a successful way, is the key, for prevention and control of HPV infections and cervical cancer.

Proposed strategy:
Knowledge transformation through p6 pathway©

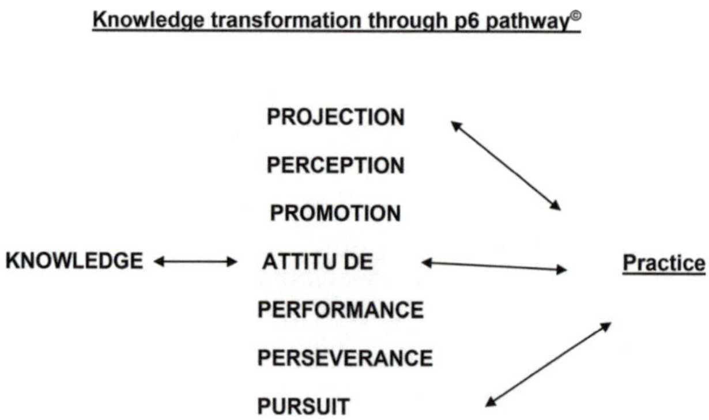

15. The P6 principles

15.1 P1. Projection

15.1.1 Health education process

It is very important that all the health-related programs have a very strong foundation with the component of health education, may it be to an individual, family, or a community. The healthcare planners, administrators, and providers are responsible for developing various methods, tools, strategies for the delivery of effective health education. In some health programs, it is called information, education, communication strategies. In this process, an idea, theme, concept, facts and figures, health topics, health problems, and solutions are being projected.

15.1.2 Negative projections

These are usually warning projections. For example, tobacco products have scary pictures of lung cancers, and head and neck cancers are printed on the packs. These are meant to arouse a sense of fear and discourage the consumer from using it. But, the feelings and its effect are temporary, resulting in continued habits. The consumers may not like the "advertisement" but likes the advertised. Such "dramatic "projections," are not ideal for health education on sensitive issues like HPV.

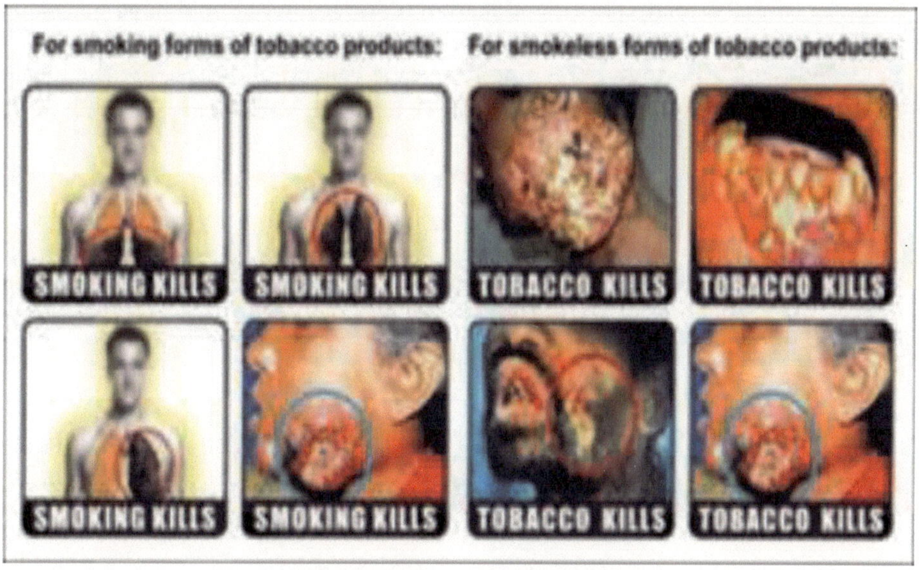

Negative projections

15.1.3 Positive/pleasant projections

The messages to be delivered are projected in a positive, attractive way. This is also a temporary appeal to their emotions. Without in-depth analysis, the consumers patronize the messages but on the long run has no permanent implications. The advertisements on the health drinks are such "positive and pleasant projections." Such projections are not suitable for behavior change targeted HP health education messages.

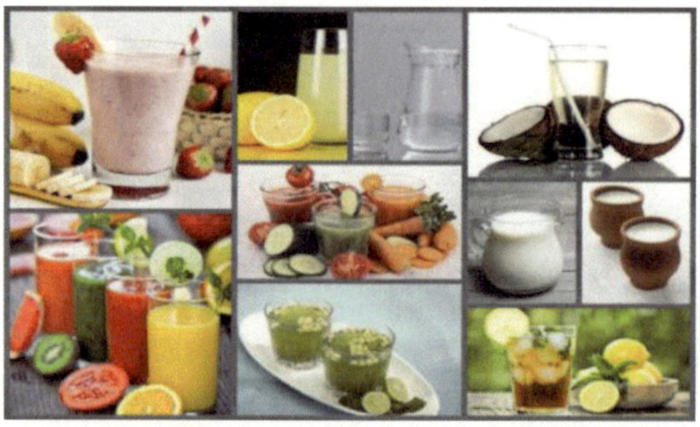

Positive/pleasant projections

15.1.4 Permanent behavior change projections

These projections are prosperous, progressive, peaceful, and productive. They imply that acceptance and adoption of the advertised message would lead to happy, healthy future. Health education messages in family planning are designed and developed like this. The example of one such advertisement shows a happy family with two children joyfully bonded with love and affection.

The consumer is highly impressed, inspired, and convinced to consider adopting family planning methods to have a small and self-sufficient family, in the future.

Likewise, in HPV-related health education messages, we should have permanent behavior change projections like HPV vaccination, menstrual hygiene, sexual hygiene, and regular periodic screening for cervix cancer, and these are the ideal and apt projections.

Permanent behavior change projections

15.1.5 The permanent behavior change projections model for HPV: cervical cancer prevention and control

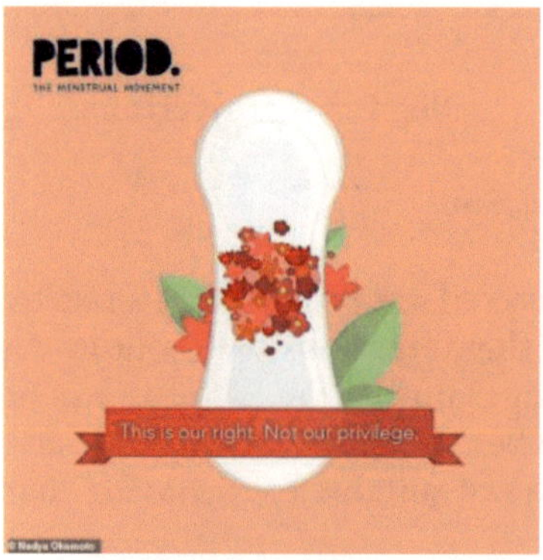
PERIOD.
THE MENSTRUAL MOVEMENT
This is our right. Not our privilege.

Menstrual hygiene

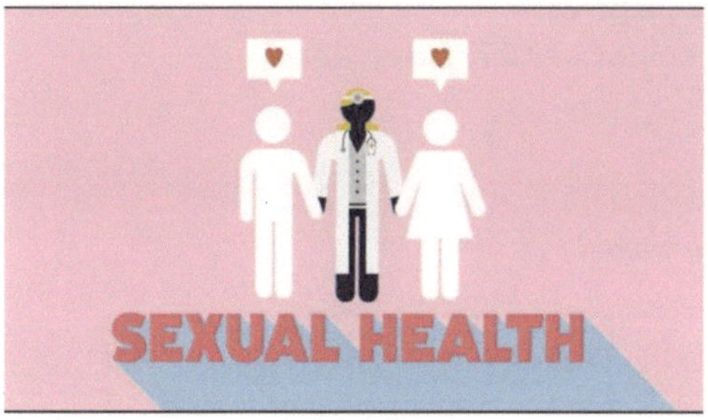

Google images Sexual hygiene

\+

HPV Vaccine

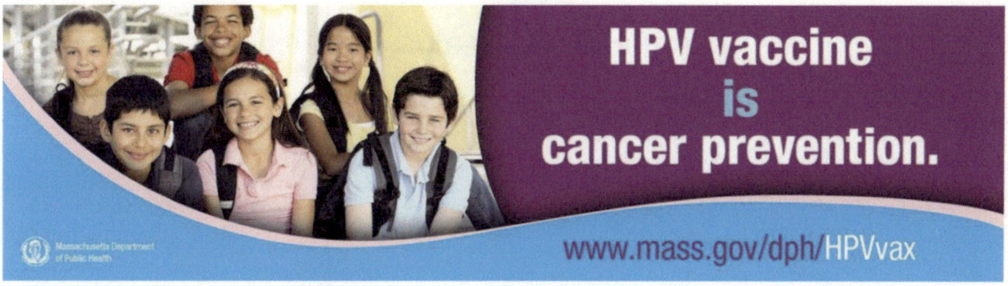

Google images

15.2 P2. Perception

It is the formation of an idea or concept, depending upon the effects of various stimuli received, to perform an act.

15.2.1 Perception process: the i5

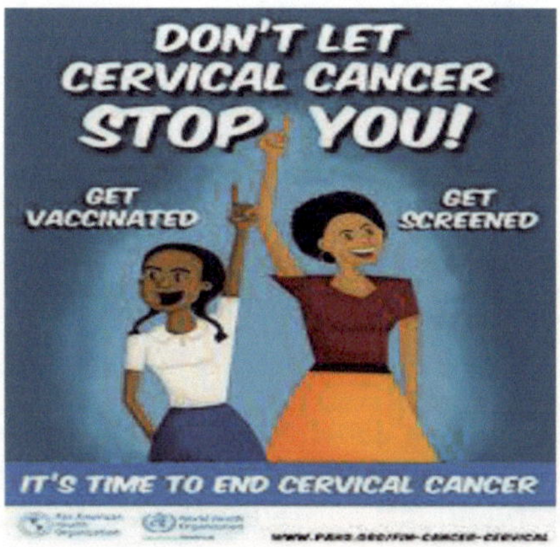

Ignite Imagine Interest Inspire Implement

Ignition: "Don't let cervical cancer stop you."
Imagine: End cervical cancer.

Interest: Easy two ways—“get vaccinated, get screened.”
Inspire: Peer group inspires.
Implement: Get vaccination/screening done.

15.3 P3. Promotion

15.3.1 Health promotion model

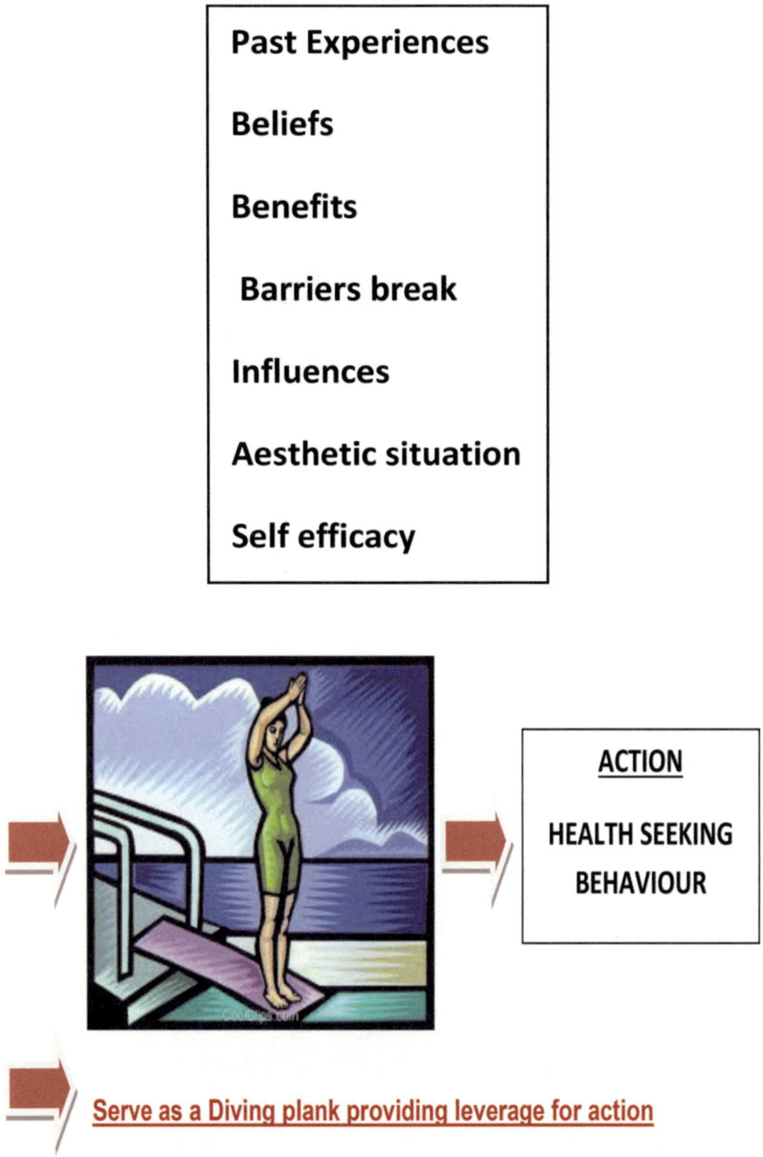

Successful and productive past experiences; beliefs getting renewed and rationalized; benefits accrued both temporarily and permanently; breaking of barriers by several inputs and interventions; positive influence from family, friends, peers, and society; esthetic situations favoring and promoting empowerment by self-efficacy, all these factors serve as a diving plank, providing strong and sustained leverage to effect “action.”

15.4 P4. Performance

15.4.1 Performance

This is a continuous process where each step is evaluated and replanned for better implementation in the next step.

Therefore in every performance, there is a betterment of the next practice. This is depicted in the performance enhancement cycle (PEC).

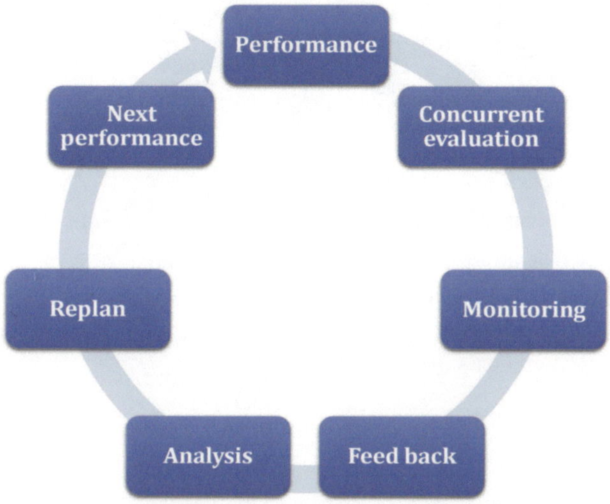

Performance enhancement cycle (PEC)

15.5 P5. Perseverance

Perseverance is constant, continued efforts and attempts, amidst of many difficulties, until the desired goal is achieved. This is an important process in healthcare delivery, where the health providers make sustained efforts to convince the healthcare recipients to adopt the desired behavior in order to achieve the appropriate and relevant goals. The act of "perseverance" largely depends upon the level and depth of perception of the health problem; the support given by family, peers, and society; and the evaluation of the eventual results and benefits. In the community, we can see the example of a pregnant woman in a family, where everyone realizes the preciousness of pregnancy and has in-depth perception and the family, relatives, community, and society offer all the support needed for the pregnant woman, amidst of many problems and difficulties, for a long period of maternity, and these acts of perseverance eventually result in the successful outcome of a safe delivery, healthy mother, and a healthy child.

In HPV control measures, perseverance is needed for effecting behavioral changes like menstrual hygiene, sexual health, adoption of HPV vaccine and most importantly screening and treatment for precancer status and regular follow-up as needed. Hence,"perseverance" in health education, healthcare delivery, and follow-up is a very important component of the goal-oriented system.

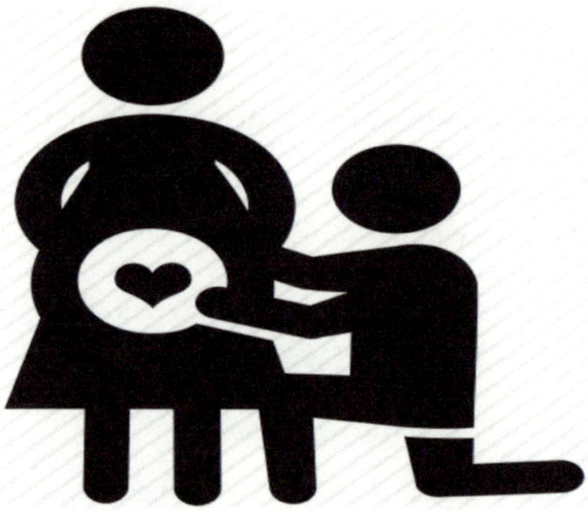

Perseverance in care during pregnancy for safe delivery

The common example of a pregnant woman and her family, community, and society, being offered all support and help for a successful outcome, amidst many difficulties, by acts of perseverance.

15.6 P6. Pursuit

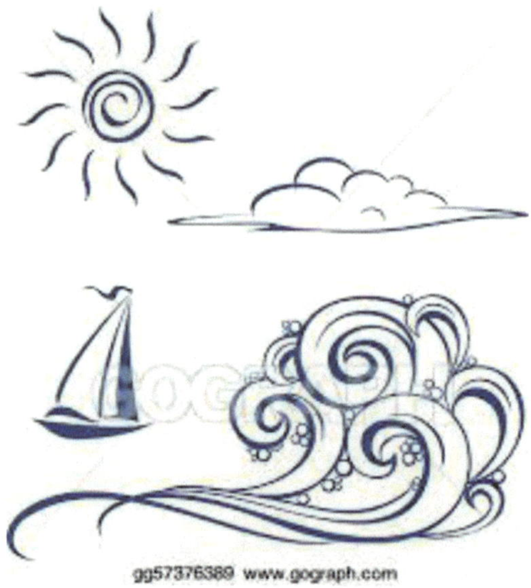

The yacht in pursuit of destination amidst problems

In pursuit of excellence is a requirement by one and all for success and achievements. In the field of healthcare planning, delivery, and implementation, one is in pursuit of excellence in technologies, techniques, strategies, skills, and scientific—social achievements.

Goals, objectives, and indicators to reach are already fixed, defined, and targeted, in a well-planned health program. The health providers are in "pursuit" of attaining these goals. There would be many difficulties, obstacles, shortcomings, and hurdles in the entire process. But, the goal is clear, and all efforts are made to overcome these, and the aim is ultimately achieved. The yacht travel which overcomes all difficulties like the sun, rain, storm, and many others, to reach its destination safely, and it's a symbolism of "pursuit."

In the HPV control programs, many such draw backs are seen. For example, illiteracy, ignorance, and poverty, prevent the usage of sanitary napkins. This is overcome by health education and mobilization of resources. The HPV vaccine has obstacles like differing policies, cost of the vaccine, lack of infrastructure to reach the vaccine to the community, and illiteracy and ignorance among the target groups. Screening programs suffer from problems like ignorant community; lack of infrastructure; deficient manpower; nonavailability of techniques, technology, and technicians; and inadequate, inefficient systems in place. Yet, these can be overcome by appropriate and adequate inputs, during the process of pursuit towards the goals by the health planners.

The health programs in the developing world do experience this act of pursuit to achieve goals, and already the results have been seen in reducing the incidence of HPV infections and cervical cancer, especially in the low and limited resource settings of many countries.

16. Raj's cancer control clock

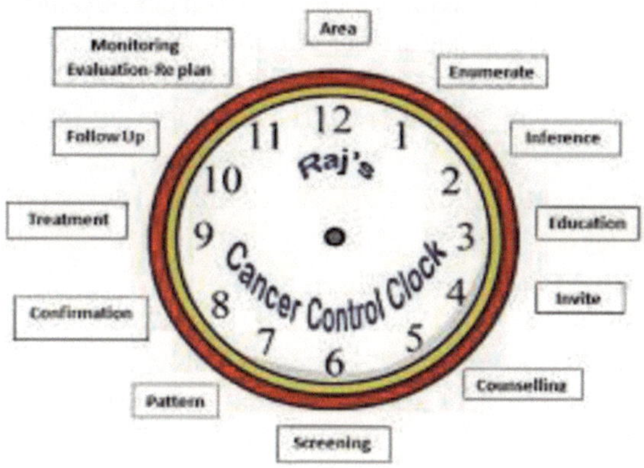

A complimentary model

The Keys for the Cancer Control Clock's 12 hours [20]:

1. **Area**—define a geographic area for your study/services

2. **Enumerate**—the resident population, document the sociodemographic data

3. **Inference**—prevalence of HPV-related diseases—establish registries

4. **Education**—about prevention at individual, family, and community levels

5. **Invitation**—to attend awareness programs, screening, and vaccination

6. **Counseling**—the participants about possible outcomes and solutions

7. **Screening**—acceptable, available, accessible, affordable, answerable, achievable—the **A-6** model for screening and vaccination programs

8. **Patterns**—of diseases detected in screening—disclosure of results—individualized, ensure confidentiality and offer solution for health problems

9. **Confirmation**—diagnosis—at screening and follow-up stages

10. **Treatment**—of the HPV infections and related diseases, precancer lesions, and ensure the availability of posttreatment services

11. **Follow-up**—by confirmation of disease free status, counseling, and referrals to the government/private health systems

12. **Monitoring, evaluation, replan**—effectiveness of interventions, health economics,and advocating prevention policies

17. Conclusion

The problem of high incidence of HPV infections and cervical cancer, all over the world, especially in developing countries is of great concern and warrants immediate control measures. Many programs have been planned and implemented and they all show promising outcomes. The HPV vaccine uptake has increased due to various inputs in developing countries. The increased vaccine coverage has shown reduced incidence of cervical precancers in longitudinal studies. The screening programs for cervical cancer have resulted in reduction in the incidence rate of cervical cancer and mortality due to cervical cancer.

18. The STAR model P-6 principles of raj©

This is a time-tested concept of the author, which was found to be very successful in the proof of concept project quoted earlier. Hence, for effective implementation of HPV and cervical cancer screening programs, especially in the phase of translating knowledge into practice, the above model is recommended, for the benefit of health programs in developing countries.

Acknowledgements

The author thankfully acknowledges Google images for the diagrams used in this paper. Immense thanks and gratitude to Celin Rani, Rijula Raj, Rixon Raj, Pavith Raj, and the angel Helena Raj, for their limitless love and care which enabled me to write this chapter. My sincere thanks to Ms. Marina Dusevic, InTech, for her masterly inputs and expert guidance, which greatly encouraged me to write this chapter. My whole-hearted thanks to the **InTech publishers**, with whom I am **editing this fifth book of mine**, for their scholastic contributions, enabling socio-scientific achievements, in the field of HPV and cervical cancer prevention, all around the globe in general and developing countries, in particular.

DOI: http://dx.doi.org/10.5772/intechopen.91313

Author details

Rajamanickam Rajkumar
Meenakshi Medical College Hospital and Research Institute of MAHER, Kanchipuram, Tamil Nadu, India

*Address all correspondence to: rajcfchc@gmail.com

References

[1] Tripathy RM, Karmee N, Behera K, Sahoo SK. Awareness and attitude about carcinoma cervix and human papillomavirus vaccine: A cross-sectional study among undergraduate female medical students. International Journal of Medical Science and Public Health. 2018;**7**(2):80-85

[2] ICO Information Centre on HPV and Cancer. Human Papillomavirus and Related Diseases in India (Summary Report 2014-08-22); 2014

[3] International Agency for Research on Cancer. IARC monographs on the evaluation of carcinogenic risks to humans. Human Papilloma Virus. Vol. 90. Lyon: International Agency for Research on Cancer; 2007

[4] Bhatla N, Lal N, Bao YP, et al. A meta-analysis of human papillomavirus type-distribution in women from South Asia: Implications for vaccination. Vaccine. 2008;**26**(23):2811-2817

[5] Moscicki AB. Impact of HPV infection in adolescent populations. The Journal of Adolescent Health. 2005;**37** (Suppl 6):S3-S9

[6] Bosch FX, Manos M, Muñoz N, et al. Prevalence of human papillomavirus in cervical cancer: A worldwide perspective. International biological study on cervical cancer study group. Journal of the National Cancer Institute. 1995;**87**(11):796-802

[7] Paavonen J. Human papillomavirus infection and the development of cervical cancer and related genital neoplasias. International Journal of Infectious Diseases. 2007;**11**(Suppl 2): S3-S9

[8] Department of Health and Human Services. Centers for disease control and prevention. Genital HPV infection fact sheet. 2004. Available from: http://www.cdc.gov/std/hpv/stdfact-hpv.htm [Accessed: 07 September 2013]

[9] Brown DR, Shew ML, Qadari B, et al. A longitudinal study of genital pappilomavirus infection in a cohort of closely followed adolescent women. The Journal of Infectious Diseases. 2006;**191**: 182-192

[10] Jacobs MV, Walboomers JM, Snijders PJ, et al. Distribution of 37 mucosotropic HPV types in women with cytologically normal cervical smears: The age-related patterns for high-risk and low-risk types. International Journal of Cancer. 2000;**87**:221-227

[11] Taylor CA, Keller ML, Egan JJ. Advice from affected persons about living with human papilloma virus infection. Image – the Journal of Nursing Scholarship. 1997;**29**(1):27-32

[12] IARC Monographs on the Evaluation of Carcinogenic Risks to Humans. Human Papilloma Viruses. Vol. 90. Lyon: International agency for research on cancer; 2006

[13] Ho GY, Bierman R, Beardsley L, Chang CJ, Burk RD. Natural history of cervicovaginal papilloma virus infection in young women. The New England Journal of Medicine. 1998;**338**: 423-428

[14] Denny L. Cervical cancer: Prevention and treatment. Discovery Medicine. 2012;**14**:125-131

[15] Hakama M, Miller AB, Day NE. Screening for Cancer of the Uterine Cervix (IARC Scientific Publications No 76). Lyon, France: IARC Press; 1986

[16] Denny L, Sankaranarayanan R. Secondary prevention of cervical cancer. International Journal of

Gynaecology and Obstetrics. 2006;**94** (Suppl 1):S65-S70

[17] Hakama M, Rasanen-Virtanen U. Effectiveness of mass screening program on the risk of cervical cancer. American Journal of Epidemiology. 1989;**17**:173-204

[18] Alliance for Cervical Cancer Prevention (ACCP). Planning and Implementing Cervical Cancer Prevention and Control Programs: A Manual for Managers. Seattle, WA, USA: ACCP; 2004

[19] Seema P, Paul B, Boffetta P. Meta analysis of social inequality and the risk of cervical cancer. International Journal of Cancer. 2003;**105**:687-691

[20] Rajamanickam Rajkumar (July 13th 2016). Introductory chapter: Human Papillomavirus (HPV) Infections, Associated Diseases and Cervical Cancer Prevention and Control Initiate Countdown Using "The Raj's Cancer Control Clock", Human Papillomavirus - Research in a Global Perspective, Rajamanickam Rajkumar, IntechOpen, DOI: 10.5772/63488. Available from: https://www.intechopen.com/books/human-papillomavirus-research-in-a-global-perspective/introductory-chapter-human-papillomavirus-hpv-infections-associated-diseases-and-cervical-cancer-pre